Differential Diagnosis
in Spine Surgery

Differential Diagnosis in Spine Surgery

Editors

John D Koerner MD
New Jersey Spinal Medicine and Surgery
Maywood, Glen Rock, New Jersey
Department of Orthopedic Surgery
Hackensack University Medical Center
Hackensack, New Jersey, USA

Alexander R Vaccaro MD PhD MBA
President, Rothman Institute
Professor and Chairman
Department of Orthopedic Surgery
Professor of Neurosurgery
Thomas Jefferson University
Philadelphia, Pennsylvania, USA

Daniel H Kim MD FAANS FACS
Professor, Director of Spinal Neurosurgery
Reconstructive Peripheral Nerve Surgery
Director of Microsurgical Robotic Lab.
Department of Neurosurgery
University of Texas
Houston, Texas, USA

Foreword
Kern Singh MD

JAYPEE *The Health Sciences Publisher*
Philadelphia | New Delhi | London | Panama

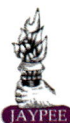 **Jaypee Brothers Medical Publishers (P) Ltd**

Headquarters
Jaypee Brothers Medical Publishers (P) Ltd.
4838/24, Ansari Road, Daryaganj
New Delhi 110 002, India
Phone: +91-11-43574357
Fax: +91-11-43574314
E-mail: jaypee@jaypeebrothers.com

Overseas Offices

J.P. Medical Ltd.
83, Victoria Street, London
SW1H 0HW (UK)
Phone: +44-20 3170 8910
Fax: +44(0)20 3008 6180
E-mail: info@jpmedpub.com

Jaypee Medical Inc.
325 Chestnut Street
Suite 412
Philadelphia, PA 19106, USA
Phone: +1 267-519-9789
E-mail: support@jpmedus.com

Jaypee-Highlights Medical Publishers Inc.
City of Knowledge, Bld. 235, 2nd Floor, Clayton
Panama City, Panama
Phone: +1 507-301-0496
Fax: +1 507-301-0499
E-mail: cservice@jphmedical.com

Jaypee Brothers Medical Publishers (P) Ltd.
17/1-B, Babar Road, Block-B, Shaymali
Mohammadpur, Dhaka-1207
Bangladesh
Mobile: +08801912003485
E-mail: jaypeedhaka@gmail.com

Jaypee Brothers Medical Publishers (P) Ltd.
Bhotahity, Kathmandu, Nepal
Phone: +977-9741283608
E-mail: kathmandu@jaypeebrothers.com

Website: www.jaypeebrothers.com
Website: www.jaypeedigital.com

Inquiries for bulk sales may be solicited at: jaypee@jaypeebrothers.com

Differential Diagnosis in Spine Surgery

First Edition: **2016**

ISBN: 978-93-85999-47-5

Printed at: Sanat Printers

Dedication

I dedicate this book to my parents
for their encouragement and support.

John D Koerner

I dedicate this book to my three children Alex, Juliana and Christian.
They are my heart and soul and the reason I enjoy the work we do in
educating future generations of spinal care physicians.

Alexander R Vaccaro

I dedicate this book to my wife Anslie and
my children Elise, Rebecca, Sarah and Isaiah.

Daniel H Kim

Contributors

Ahmed J Awad MD
Department of Neurosurgery
Icahn School of Medicine at
Mount Sinai
Mount Sinai Health System
New York, New York, USA
Faculty of Medicine and
Health Sciences
An-Najah National University
Nablus, Palestine

Caleb Behrend MD
Carilion Clinic Orthopedics
Assistant Professor
Department of Orthopedic Surgery
Virginia Tech Carilion
School of Medicine
Roanoke, Virginia, USA

Tamir Bloom MD
Advocare Orthopedics
Cedar Knolls, New Jersey
Adjunct Professor
Department of Orthopedics
Rutgers University—New Jersey
Medical School
Newark, New Jersey, USA

Brian P Calio BA
Thomas Jefferson University
Sidney Kimmel Medical College
Philadelphia, Pennsylvania, USA

Angela Chang BS
Drexel University College of Medicine
Philadelphia, Pennsylvania, USA

Saad B Chaudhary MD MBA
Minimally Invasive and Complex
Spine Surgery
Assistant Professor
Icahn School of Medicine at
Mount Sinai
Department of Orthopedic Surgery
Mount Sinai Beth Israel
New York, New York, USA

Tim Colangelo BA
Drexel University College of Medicine
Philadelphia, Pennsylvania, USA

Mike Donahue MD
Clinical Associate Professor
Michigan State University
East Lansing, Michigan, USA

Adam E Flanders MD
Department of Radiology
Division of Neuroradiology/ENT
Thomas Jefferson University Hospital
Philadelphia, Pennsylvania, USA

Tristan Fried BS
Thomas Jefferson University
Sidney Kimmel Medical College
Philadelphia, Pennsylvania, USA

George M Ghobrial MD
Department of Neurosurgery
Thomas Jefferson University
Philadelphia, Pennsylvania, USA

Stephanie Wrobel Goldberg MD
Headache Fellow
Thomas Jefferson University Hospital
Philadelphia, Pennsylvania, USA

Matthew Goldfarb BS
Thomas Jefferson University
Sidney Kimmel Medical College
Philadelphia, Pennsylvania, USA

Martin Griffis BA, MS
Drexel University College of Medicine
Philadelphia, Pennsylvania, USA

James S Harrop MD
Professor of Neurosurgery
Director, Division of Spine and
Peripheral Nerve Disorders
Thomas Jefferson University
Philadelphia, Pennsylvania, USA

Kevin Henrichsen MD
Thomas Jefferson University
Sidney Kimmel Medical College
Philadelphia, Pennsylvania, USA

Heidi M Hullinger MD
Clinical Assistant Professor of
Orthopedics
Rutgers University—New Jersey
Medical School
Newark, New Jersey, USA

Daniel H Kim MD FAANS FACS
Professor
Director of Spinal Neurosurgery
Reconstructive Peripheral
Nerve Surgery
Director of Microsurgical Robotic Lab.
Department of Neurosurgery
University of Texas
Houston, Texas, USA

John D Koerner MD
New Jersey Spinal
Medicine and Surgery
Maywood, Glen Rock, New Jersey
Department of Orthopedic Surgery
Hackensack University Medical Center
Hackensack, New Jersey, USA

Rex AW Marco MD
Associate Professor of
Orthopedic Surgery
Institute for Academic Medicine
Houston Methodist Hospital
Weill Cornell Medical College
Houston, Texas, USA

Christopher M Maulucci MD
Department of Neurosurgery
Thomas Jefferson University
Philadelphia, Pennsylvania, USA

Loren Mead BA
Spine Research Fellow
Rothman Institute
Philadelphia, Pennsylvania, USA

Saint-Aaron Morris MD
Department of Neurosurgery
University of Texas Health
Science Center
Houston, Texas, USA

Troy Mounts MD
Orthopedic Spine Surgeon
French Hospital Medical Center
San Luis Obispo, California, USA

Sarah Nyirjesy BA
Drexel University College of Medicine
Philadelphia, Pennsylvania, USA

Andrew G Park MD
Department of Orthopedic Surgery
Thomas Jefferson University
Philadelphia, Pennsylvania, USA

Sanjeev Sabharwal MD MPH
Professor, Orthopedic Surgery
Rutgers University—New Jersey
Medical School
Newark, New Jersey, USA

Alexander J Schupper BA
UC San Diego School of Medicine
San Diego, California, USA

Karim Shafi BS
Thomas Jefferson University
Sidney Kimmel Medical College
Philadelphia, Pennsylvania, USA

Anuj Shah BA
Thomas Jefferson University
Sidney Kimmel Medical College
Philadelphia, Pennsylvania, USA

Stephen Silberstein MD
Director Jefferson Headache Center
Thomas Jefferson University
Philadelphia, Pennsylvania, USA

Jessica Stark MD
Department of Neurosurgery
University of Texas
Houston, Texas, USA

Christie Stawicki BA
Spine Research Fellow
Rothman Institute
Philadelphia, Pennsylvania, USA

Alexander R Vaccaro MD PhD MBA
President, Rothman Institute
Richard H Rothman
Professor and Chairman
Department of Orthopedic Surgery
Professor of Neurosurgery
Thomas Jefferson University
Philadelphia, Pennsylvania, USA

Colin Vroome MD
Thomas Jefferson University
Sidney Kimmel Medical College
Philadelphia, Pennsylvania, USA

Brett Walker MD
Clinical Associate Professor
Michigan State University
East Lansing, Michigan, USA

Vahe M Zohrabian MD
Assistant Professor of Radiology and
Biomedical Imaging
Yale Medical School
New Haven, Connecticut, USA

Foreword

Spinal disorders are among the most common reasons patients present to clinicians. The differential diagnosis for these pathologies includes a wide spectrum of disorders encompassing multiple organ systems. Being able to thoroughly and efficiently evaluate patients is imperative for the busy clinician. This book provides a systematic approach to patients presenting with the most common spine and non-spine related disorders. In addition, this textbook details the appropriate workup for less commonly evaluated pathologies and their clinical nuances. Clearly, this treatise provides essential information for trainees as well as the experienced clinician in handling spinal and non-spinal pathologies.

Kern Singh MD
Associate Professor
Department of Orthopedic Surgery
Rush University Medical Center
Co-Director
Minimally Invasive Spine Institute at Rush
Chicago, Illinois, USA

Preface

Neck and back pain are among the most common reasons patients seek medical attention. Evaluating these issues in an efficient and thorough manner are key for the busy clinician. This book describes some of the most common reasons patients with spinal pathology present to physicians, and explains the differential diagnosis and appropriate workup for each condition. The most common diagnoses are described in detail, along with red-flags to be aware of. The spine clinician should be aware of non-spine pathologies that may present with neck or back pain, and how to initiate the appropriate workup. This book will be helpful to spine and non-spine clinicians in reaching a diagnosis for patients presenting with neck and back related complaints.

John D Koerner MD
Alexander R Vaccaro MD PhD MBA
Daniel H Kim MD FAANS FACS

Acknowledgments

We would like to thank Mr Jitendar P Vij (Group Chairman), Mr Ankit Vij (Group President), Ms Chetna Malhotra Vohra (Associate Director), Ms Angima Shree (Senior Development Editor), and the production team of Jaypee Brothers Medical Publishers (P) Ltd, New Delhi, India.

Contents

CHAPTER 1

Lower Back Pain in Children and Adolescents

Tamir Bloom, Sanjeev Sabharwal, Saad B Chaudhary

INTRODUCTION

Lower back pain is uncommon in young children (< 10 years old) but may be experienced by as many as 36% of older children and adolescents,[1,2] with an even higher incidence in competitive adolescent athletes.[3-5] In the older child or adolescent, the evaluation of nonspecific, chronic back pain (lasting > 3 months) frequently does not result in an identifiable organic cause despite the use of an extensive diagnostic workup.[6] While young children are more likely to have an underlying pathologic cause for their discomfort, mechanical back pain (defined as pain when there is no identifiable etiology detected on physical examination, radiographs, or advanced imaging investigation) accounts for the majority of juvenile and adolescent lower back pain.[6-9] It is important to be able to discern patients who have mechanical back pain, and require only symptomatic treatment and observation, from patients with a suspected serious organic cause for the symptoms so that sophisticated diagnostic imaging studies and laboratory tests can be appropriately obtained and timely treatment can be instituted. The initial step in differentiating between patients who experience mechanical back pain from those with a specific etiology or demonstrable pathology is a careful medical history and a physical examination.

CHIEF COMPLAINT/HISTORY

A thorough history provides the clinician with the most vital diagnostic tool when evaluating a child with lower back pain. Furthermore, a comprehensive clinical assessment, with interview questions based on pertinent differential diagnosis can help direct further workup. Perform the initial history with the parents present and in methodical fashion. Have patients describe the nature of their pain including, location (symmetric or asymmetric, midline or paraspinal), nature of onset, character (dull, aching, or sharp), severity, timing, frequency, and any associated radiation. It may be challenging to get children to answer all questions accurately as they are not always specific in localizing the area of concern. The interaction between the patient and the parents may provide clues as to their relationship and may shed light on the nature of the child's pain. Any changes or limitations in the child's activity because of pain can help to understand the severity of the pain. The clinician should also inquire about any history of prior trauma, aggravating and alleviating factors, the presence of neurological symptoms, changes in the child's gait or posture, constitutional symptoms, history of prior infection, including any systemic illness. In young athletes, questions related to sports, including the type of activities, amount of training per day or week, type of training, amount of training per year (down-time) for specific sports, supervision of training, and expectations or importance of that particular sport to both the athlete and the family can provide insightful information.[10,11]

Lower back pain is a relatively common complaint in the skeletally immature patient, and the following generalizations may help in identifying children with a diagnosable pathology. Commonly, an underlying cause for back pain is found in children whose duration of pain is greater than 4 weeks but less than 3 months.[7] Young children and toddlers who present with pain are unlikely to exaggerate symptoms or physical findings, and frequently have a specific pathologic process causing their symptoms. Warning signs where an underlying abnormality is likely to be found include persistent or increasing pain, being worse at night or when lying down, radicular pain, neurologic deficits, loss of motion, spasms, and systemic symptoms (Box 1.1).[9] Identifying spinal cord or nerve root impingement requires understanding of neurological symptoms, such as radiculopathy, myelopathy, gait changes, and bowel or bladder changes.

Nonspecific back pain in teenagers may be associated with psychosocial factors (e.g. increasing difficulty with school performance, social maladjustment, physical/sexual abuse, teen pregnancy, and recent familial unrest/death/divorce) or psychological problems (e.g. anxiety disorders, depression, and attempted suicide), as well as litigation and psychosomatic conversion reaction. When appropriate, inquire about family members or friends with similar symptoms and whether they have any disability or physical handicaps. In our experience, a child with back pain related to a history of a motor vehicle accident, whether recent or remote often have lingering back pain. Inquire about a possible history of litigation and be wary when the parents do not allow the child to directly respond to physician's questions.

History regarding backpack wear and the amount of weight within the backpack,[12-15] as well as amount of time playing video games[16] and tobacco use[17,18] should be discussed as these have also been implicated in nonspecific lower back pain in adolescence. In addition, medical history, medications, surgical history, and family history may provide insight to other causes of pain or possible predisposing reasons for pain.

> **Box 1.1:** Pediatric lower back pain history: Pertinent red flags.
>
> - Pain in a young child, especially if they stop playing or unexplained refusal to walk
> - Pain at rest (not including pain with sitting; pain with prolonged sitting in school that is relieved by lying down is extremely common in teenagers with mechanical low back pain)
> - Pain that is unrelenting, getting worse, or is not relieved by nonsteroidal anti-inflammatory medication
> - Radicular pain
> - Night pain
> - Change or loss of bowel or bladder control
> - Pain with urination, defecation, coughing or sneezing
> - Recurrent urinary tract infection
> - Worsening spasticity, progressive weakness, rapidly increasing scoliosis
> - Constitutional symptoms (fever, chills, lethargy, weight loss, loss of appetite, malaise)

DIFFERENTIAL DIAGNOSIS

Although no condition is exclusive to a particular age group, the age of the patient is helpful in establishing a differential diagnosis (Table 1.1). Children below the age of 4 years are more likely to have infection or neoplasm, whereas mechanical back pain or pain associated with trauma or overuse syndromes is more often encountered in patients greater than 10 years. Characteristics of the pain (onset, duration, timing, and location) offer valuable information. In general, patients with mechanical back pain present with complaints of non-neurologic, nonspecific, intermittent and chronic pain. Pain of sudden onset or pain that is most intense 24–48 hours after injury, heavy lifting, or vigorous physical activity occurs commonly from self-limited lumbar sprains or strains, or less frequently from a fracture, apophyseal ring injury, or herniated disk. The most common identifiable diagnosis producing lumbar back pain in active patients between the ages of 10 and 15 years is spondylolysis or spondylolisthesis.[19] Painful defects, fractures, and stress lesions within the pars interarticularis are often seen in patients participating in sports that tend to involve repetitive hyperextension of the spine, such as gymnastics, figure skating, cheerleading, football (linemen), and volleyball. Athletes involved in these particular sports may also develop pain secondary to degenerative disk disease, but exact correlation between a degenerative intervertebral disk and lower back pain remains elusive.[20] Insidious pain that is activity related and relieved with rest may also be due to recurrent lumbar strains/sprains, spondylolysis, apophyseal ring fractures, and sacral stress fractures.

Persistent lower back pain not associated with trauma and not relieved by 2–3 weeks rest, activity modification, nonsteroidal anti-inflammatories, or pain that awakens the patient from sleep is more concerning for infection

Table 1.1: Differential diagnosis of common spinal causes of pediatric lower back pain (LBP) by age.

	Presenting characteristics of lower back pain	Associated symptoms
Birth to 4 years		
Diskitis/osteomyelitis	• Nonspecific • Unremitting, night pain	• Limp, hip or leg pain (refusal to walk) • Abdominal pain • Systemic symptoms (fever, poor appetite, lethargy, malaise)
Malignant tumors (e.g. leukemia, lymphoma, sarcoma) Metastases to the spine (e.g. neuroblastoma, rhabdomyosarcoma) Tumor-like lesions (e.g. eosinophilic granuloma)	• Slow-onset, nonspecific LBP • Progressively more severe • Unrelenting • Night pain	• Radiating pain below the knees • Systemic symptoms
5–11 years		
Diskitis/osteomyelitis	• Nonspecific • Unremitting, night pain	• Limp, hip or leg pain (refusal to walk) • Systemic symptoms
Benign bone tumors (e.g. osteoid osteoma, osteoblastoma) Bone cyst (unicameral or aneurysmal)	• Slow-onset • Sharp, constant • Worse at night • Alleviated by NSAIDs	
Malignant tumors and metastases (e.g.osteosarcoma, Ewing's sarcoma) Spinal cord tumors (e.g. astrocytoma, ependymoma)	• Nonspecific • Unremitting, night pain	• Systemic symptoms • Gait abnormalities, delay in achieving motor milestones
Idiopathic juvenile osteoporosis	• Extreme pain	• Difficulty walking
12 years to maturity		
Mechanical back pain	• Chronic or intermittent • Nonspecific • Aggravated by prolonged standing, walking or sitting • Alleviated by NSAIDs, rest, massage, heat	• No radicular symptoms
Muscle strain/ligament strain	• Acute, short duration • Sharp, mild • Alleviated by NSAIDs, rest, massage, heat	• Muscle tenderness without radiation

Contd…

Contd…

	Presenting characteristics of lower back pain	*Associated symptoms*
Spondylolysis/ spondylolisthesis	• Acute or chronic • Dull or aching • Intermittent or recurrent • Aggravated by sports, particularly those involving repetitive hyperextension of the trunk • Relieved by rest or restriction of athletic or physical activity, NSAIDs	• Pain radiating to gluteal region and posterior thighs • Spasms of paravertebral or hamstring muscles • Bowel or bladder dysfunction can occur with significant slip progression • Lumbar or thoracolumbar scoliosis may occur with spondylolisthesis
Herniated intervertebral disk	• Acute or insidious • Insidious, recurrent or with activity • Aggravated by prolonged walking or sitting, coughing or sneezing • Alleviated by NSAIDs, rest, massage, heat	• Radicular pain to the buttock, lateral thigh, or leg
Slipped vertebral ring apophysis	• Acute, sharp, constant • Aggravated by prolonged walking or sitting, coughing or sneezing • Alleviated by NSAIDs, rest	• Radicular pain to the buttock or lateral thigh, usually bilateral
Degenerative disk disease	• Chronic • Activity related • Alleviated by NSAIDs, rest, massage, heat	• Spasms of paravertebral or hamstring muscles
Ankylosing spondylitis, other spondyloarthritides	• Insidious, slow-onset, chronic (> 3 months) • Dull or achy • Pain and stiffness usually worse in the mornings and during the night, may improve by warm shower or light exercise but not with rest	• Morning stiffness • Joint pain, swelling of the lower limbs • Symptoms of anterior uveitis (eye redness, pain, light sensitivity, vision problems, etc.) • Constitutional symptoms
Lumbar Scheuermann's kyphosis	• Slow-onset, chronic • Dull or achy • Aggravated by prolonged sitting, walking or activity	
Infection—diskitis, vertebral (pyogenic) osteomyelitis, tuberculous spondylitis (non-pyogenic)	• Slow-onset, may be chronic for non-pyogenic infection • Dull, achy, or sharp • Aggravated by activity, may also include night and resting pain	• Limp, hip or leg pain • Abdominal pain • Systemic symptoms

Contd…

Contd…

	Presenting characteristics of lower back pain	Associated symptoms
Sacralization of L5/ transverse process impingement Bertolotti's syndrome[21]	• Chronic • Dull or achy • Activity related	• Chronic sciatica
Psychogenic back pain, conversion reactions	• Slow-onset, chronic • Dull or achy	
Tumors of the spine	• Unremitting, persistent • Not activity related	• Systemic symptoms

(NSAIDs: Nonsteroidal anti-inflammatory drugs).

Table 1.2: Pediatric lower back pain not localized to the lumbar spine.

Sacral and sacroiliac joint	• Sacroiliitis (associated with ankylosing spondylitis) • Pyogenic sacroiliitis • Sacral stress fracture[22] • Arachnoid cyst[23,24]
Intra-abdominal/renal	• Appendicitis • Inflammatory bowel disease • Hydronephrosis • Urinary tract infection/pyelonephritis • Gynecologic abnormalities, e.g. ovarian cysts • Psoas abscess
Diagnoses of exclusion	• Overuse syndromes • Pain associated with menstrual period • Psychosomatic (conversion reaction)

(Frymoyer, John W; Wiesel, Sam W, et al. eds. The Adult & Pediatric Spine. Chpt 21. "Back Pain in Children and Adolescents" Lippincott Williams & Wilkins. 2004).

or neoplasm. Night pain that prevents the patient from going to sleep but once asleep does not awaken the patient is more common in mechanical conditions. On the other hand, night pain, due to which the patient is awakened from sleep by the pain, is more likely to be due to a more serious condition and should always raise the concern of an infection or neoplastic condition (Table 1.2). Pain localized to the lower lumbar spine is more commonly seen in conditions such as spondylolysis and spondylolisthesis; pain in the sacroiliac (SI) area may indicate an inflammatory arthropathy, infection, or tumor. Infections and neoplasms may occur in any portion of the spinal column. Symmetric pain may be due to mechanical or an overuse condition, whereas asymmetric pain localized to one side of the spine may be more likely due to spondylolysis or tumors. Pain worsened by coughing or sneezing, radicular pain, change in bowel or bladder habits, asymmetric foot posturing or deformities may indicate the presence of conditions that can cause neural compression (e.g. herniated nucleus pulposus, intraspinal tumors, tethered spinal cord, syringomyelia, or severe spondylolisthesis).

WORKUP

Anatomy/Physical Exam

Visual Inspection and Assessment of Alignment and Motion

The physical examination of a pediatric patient should be tailored to each age group and suspected disease process. Enlisting the parents or caregivers with the examination, for example by demonstrating the exam technique first on the parent, may facilitate cooperation with the examination on a young or developmentally delayed child. A comprehensive examination should begin with placing the child in a gown (open in the back) with all articles of clothing removed, except for underpants or shorts, and long hair should be lifted so that the entire spine can be examined. Socks should be removed to look for any foot deformities that may signify intraspinal anomalies or tethered cord. Note the child's height, weight, and body habitus. Being overweight or obese is an important factor associated with back pain and can be identified by determining the body mass index (*Source*: apps.nccd.cdc.gov/dnpabmi/Calculator.aspx).[25,26]

Observe the child's gait and standing coronal and sagittal posture with both lower extremities uncovered. In young children, watching the patient walk in the hallway, entering the examination room, or playing can frequently detect abnormalities in gait, strength, posture and balance. Children with severe spondylolisthesis may have a wide-based stance with the hips and knees flexion, a stiff lumbar spine with marked lumbar hyperlordosis, associated posterior pelvic tilt, heart-shaped buttocks (owing to the vertical position of the sacrum), a protruding abdomen, and a palpable "step-off" often noted at the lumbosacral junction. This standing posture has been described as the Phalen-Dickson sign.[27] The normal heel-to-toe gait pattern may change in conditions associated with hamstring tightness, such as spondylolysis and spondylolisthesis. Hamstring tightness may prevent full extension of the knee in terminal swing (stiff-knee gait pattern), thereby causing a decrease in stride length. A limp or ataxia, with or without pain, may be the presenting sign of an intraspinal disorder.

With the child standing, inspect the back for cutaneous findings. A hair patch, subcutaneous lipoma, hemangioma, or sacral dimple may indicate spinal dysraphism. Café-au-lait spots may indicate neurofibromatosis. Assess posture and coronal and sagittal alignment for signs of scoliosis or kyphosis. When viewing a patient from a lateral position, a kyphotic deformity is evident at the thoracic spine or the thoracolumbar junction in Scheuermann's disease. The angular kyphosis is seen most clearly when the patient bends forward, distinguishing it from postural kyphosis which is flexible (Figs. 1.1A to D). Patients with Scheuermann's disease may stand with compensatory lumbar and cervical lordosis, as well as with the shoulders appearing

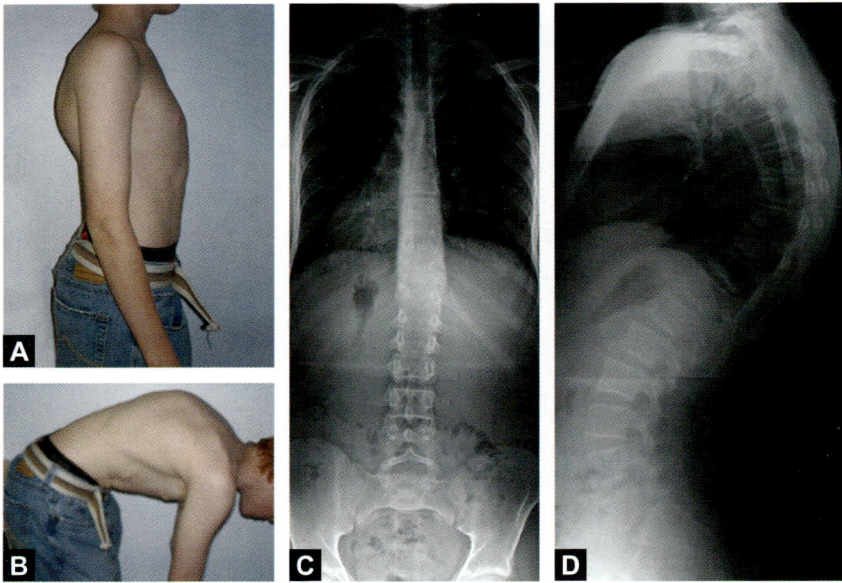

Figs. 1.1A to D: Clinical appearance of a 17-year-old male with long standing back pain and pronounced thoracic kyphosis due to Scheuermann's disease. (A) Standing sagittal alignment demonstrating greater than normal thoracic kyphosis and rounding of the shoulders, (B) With the patient bending forward, an angular kyphosis is seen rather than the normal gradual rounding of the thoracic spine, (C and D) Posteroanterior and lateral radiographs demonstrate a thoracic kyphotic deformity in the order of 85°, vertebral end plate irregularities, and the anterior vertebral wedging in the thoracic spine.

rounded and the head protruding forward. Look for any asymmetry in the neck, level of the shoulders, level of the scapular spines, prominence of the scapulae, surface of the rib cage, and contour of the flanks. The iliac crests are palpated to determine if they are level, or the posterior iliac dimples may be observed for symmetry, indicating equal leg lengths (Fig. 1.2). A difference in the level of the iliac crest may indicate a limb-length discrepancy that can cause a compensatory scoliosis deformity (convex toward the shorter limb) to balance the head over the pelvis. This postural scoliosis will disappear when the leg lengths are corrected by placing an appropriately sized lift under the foot of the short leg. A plumb line, measured by suspending a weight from a string from the C7 spinous process to the level of the pelvis, can be used to determine if the spine is compensated or decompensated. If the spine is compensated, a plumb bob should lie directly over the center of the gluteal cleft. If there is coronal decompensation, usually secondary to scoliosis, the plumb bob will fall 2 cm or more on either side of the gluteal cleft.

The Adam's forward-bending test is useful to detect scoliosis and to determine if the spine is supple and flexes symmetrically. With the clinician standing behind the patient, perform the test by having the patient bending

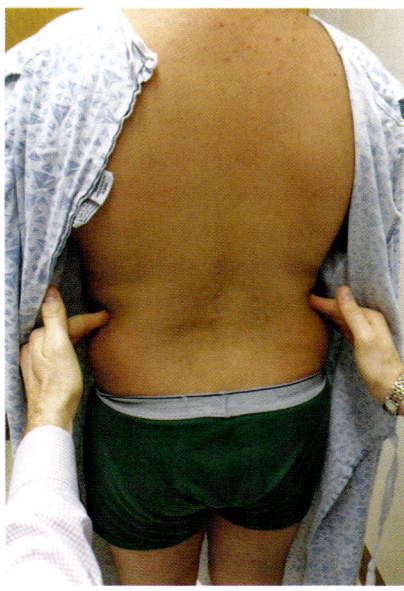

Fig. 1.2: Clinical photograph demonstrating symmetric palpation of the iliac crests indicating a level pelvis.

forward at the waist and the arms hanging freely in front with the palms opposed. Ensure that the knees are fully extended and have the patient reach for their toes. If the patient bends to one side instead of straight ahead, it may indicate a hamstring contracture. With the patient's spine parallel to the floor, asymmetry of the trunk may be observed indicating a rotational component of a scoliosis deformity (Figs. 1.3A to C). The angular degree of thoracic or lumbar prominence can be assessed using a scoliometer placed at the point of maximal asymmetry to measure the angle of trunk rotation, or rib prominence. With the spine flexed, hamstring and paraspinal tightness can be assessed by measuring the distance from the floor to the patient's fingertips. Limited forward bending may be associated with back pain and spondylolisthesis.[18] In toddlers and children, the "coin test" may indicate an inability to flex the lower back, assessed by placing an object, such as a coin (or a candy), on the floor and asking the child to pick it up. The test is positive if the back is held in an abnormally stiff posture, with the loss of the usually smooth flexion and extension of the spine, and bends primarily at the hips and knees. Toddlers or children with diskitis commonly present with a positive coin test, loss of lumbar lordosis, refusal to walk, limp, and hip or leg pain.[28] In general, pain provoked with back hyperextension and relieved with flexion is usually the result of pathology from the posterior spinal elements (pars interarticularis, facet joints, spinous processes). Pain with hyperflexion but relief in extension, arises from the vertebral bodies, disks, or anterior soft tissues. Further assess spinal mobility with extension,

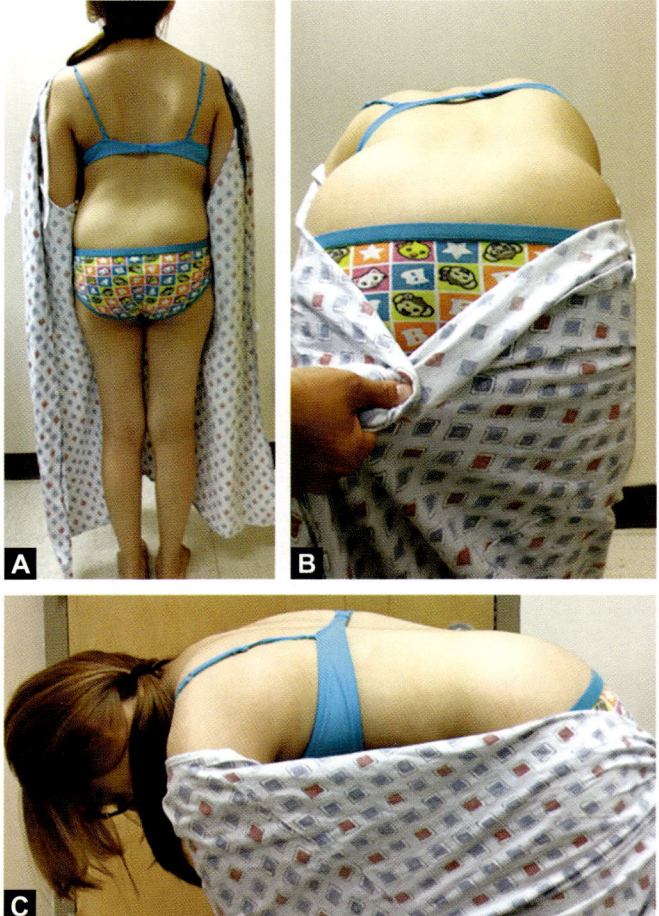

Figs. 1.3A to C: (A) Clinical photograph of a 12-year-old female demonstrating a prominent right scapula, asymmetry in the level of the shoulder, and asymmetry of the flank commonly seen in adolescent idiopathic scoliosis, (B) Adam's forward-bending test reveals one side of the back appears higher than the other, (C) The clinical appearance on the sagittal profile illustrating rib asymmetry and loss of normal thoracic kyphosis.

rotation or bending at the waist, and to the right and left, as motion may be restricted in patients with lower back pain or paraspinal muscle spasm.

Ask the child to localize the back pain with the point of a finger. A child or adolescent that points to one spot, a positive "finger test," may more likely to have true pathology causing their back pain. An adolescent with typical mechanical back pain is more likely to localize their pain over a broad area, particularly transversely across the lower back. Palpate the spinous processes and sacrum for areas of focal tenderness and percuss any areas of pain identified by the patient. Patients with spondylolysis will frequently experience pain when the affected spinous process is palpated, particularly at the L5 spinous process. Tenderness over the paraspinal muscles may indicate muscle spasms. Defects in the posterior elements may be palpated by running the fingers along the spine.

A single-leg lumbar hyperextension test (Stork test) is performed by having the patient stand on one leg with the contralateral knee flexed and hyperextending the back (Fig. 1.4). The testing position increases pressure at the pars interarticularis on the side of weight bearing. Lumbar pain on the weight-bearing side is a common finding in patients with spondylolysis or spondylolisthesis. This procedure also assesses proprioception and stability. Pain originating from the SI joint may be detected with the Patrick or Flexion, Abduction, and External Rotation (FABER) test. This test is performed with the patient lying supine, placing the foot of the affected side on the contralateral knee and pressing firmly on the flexed knee and on the opposite anterior superior iliac crest; this maneuver enhances pain localized to the SI area. Hamstring flexibility may further be assessed by measuring the popliteal angle. With the patient supine, place the contralateral leg flat on the exam table. The ipsilateral hip is flexed 90° and the knee is gradually extended to its natural limit. The angle formed by a vertical line along the posterior thigh and calf is measured. Popliteal angle less than 130° indicated hamstring tightness.[29] While lying supine, the lower extremities can be examined for equal leg lengths, joint deformity, and muscle bulk.

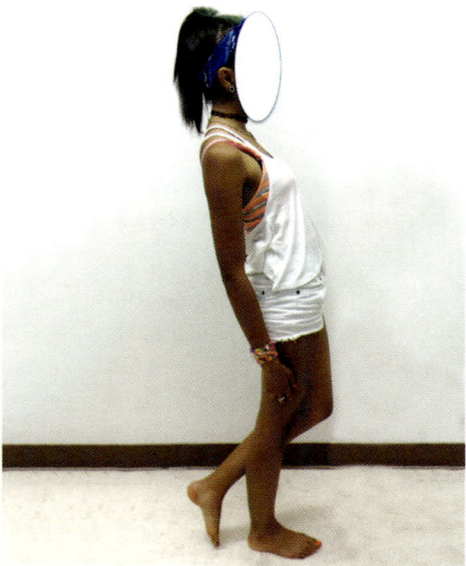

Fig. 1.4: The Stork test is performed with the patient standing on one leg and extending the lumbar spine. Pain in the lower back with hyperextension is a common finding in spondylolysis and spondylolisthesis. This test also assesses global proprioception and stability. This test can be performed with the patient's eyes closed to further assess proprioception in the absence of visual input. A positive finding is the patient's inability to stand with little or no body motion for 10 seconds.

Neurologic Examination

A thorough neurological examination of the extremities includes assessment for muscle strength, sensation, deep tendon reflexes, and presence of any long tract signs, such as muscle wasting, fasciculations, weakness, hypertonia/hypotonia, clonus, hyper-reflexia, altered or loss of sensation, and sphincter disorders (disorders of urination, bowel and sexual function). In a busy office setting, this can be accomplished efficiently by having the child heel walk, toe walk, and perform a single-leg hop on each foot in turn to assess the general strength, muscle tone and coordination. Performing a straight-leg raise test, standard lower extremity joint reflexes, abdominal reflexes, Babinski test, checking for sustained clonus, and sensory examination can evaluate for neurologic abnormalities. Adolescent lumbar disk herniation, occurring most commonly at the L5/S1 level followed by L4/L5,[30] may present with an abnormal motor, sensory, and reflex examination. A disk protrusion at L5/S1 usually affects the first sacral nerve root causing sensory changes over lateral aspects of the calf and foot, weakness in the gastrocsoleus muscle and a decreased Achilles tendon reflex. A disk protrusion at L4/L5 usually affects the L5 nerve root and may cause sensory changes over the dorsal and medial aspect of the foot, particularly the first web space, weakness in dorsiflexion of the great toe and inversion. Increased or asymmetric reflexes can indicate myelopathic or intramedullary lesions involving the spinal cord. A straight-leg raise test is important for assessing signs related to lumbar nerve root irritation. The test is performed with the patient supine, with the examiner gradually raising one leg with the hip and knee in extension. A positive test reproduces the patient's radicular symptoms with the leg elevated off the exam table. The test is reported as an angle between the lower limb and the tabletop. A contralateral straight-leg raise test should also be performed as it can function as a confirmatory test with high specificity for diagnosing a disk herniation. A positive test reproduces the patient's radicular symptoms with raising the unaffected side. Although less common, an upper lumbar disk herniation can be responsible for back pain and radiculopathy and can be aptly evaluated with a femoral stretch test. This test is generally performed with the patient in the prone position with the knee passively flexed to the thigh and the hip passively extended. Again a positive test results in reproduction of the patient's symptoms with this provocative maneuver. Assess the feet for abnormalities such as, cavus foot, clubfoot, and clawing of the digits.

Imaging Studies

The most useful imaging study in children with back pain is a standing anteroposterior (AP) and lateral radiograph of the portion of the spine that

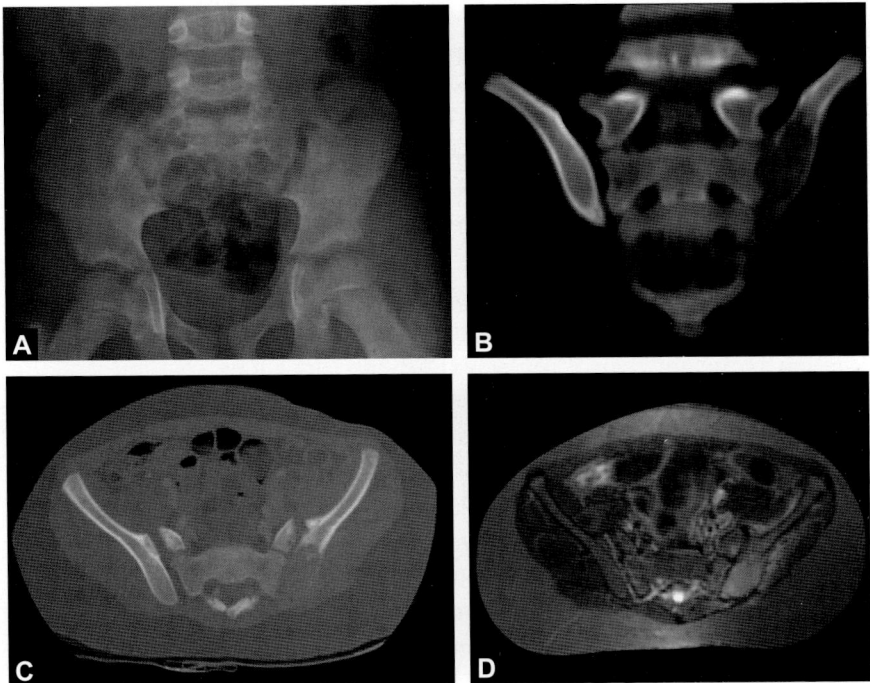

Figs. 1.5A to D: A 9-year-old boy with a history of left sacroiliac joint pain. (A) Anteroposterior radiograph of the pelvis demonstrates focal osteopenia in the left sacral ala, (B and C) Coronal and axial CT of the pelvis shows a lytic lesion destroying the posterior and medial cortex of the left ilium with disruption of the articular surface of the left ilium, (D) Axial T2-Fast Spin Echo weighted image shows the lesion extending into the sacroiliac joint with soft tissue edema. Incisional biopsy was consistent with anaplastic lymphoma.

seems to be involved, either thoracolumbar or lumbosacral spine. Consider including the pelvis, because some lesions in the pelvis and sacrum, e.g. osteoid osteoma and spinal arachnoid cysts, may cause lower back pain (Figs. 1.5A to D). Lead-shielding to minimize ionizing radiation exposure to the gonads should not be used for the initial radiographs because it may obscure a lesion in this region. Radiographs should be obtained during the initial evaluation of all children (age 10 years or younger) with persistent, unremitting lower back pain longer than 6 weeks, or who have any "red flags" (*see* Box 1.1). On the AP image, evaluate for normal vertebral body morphology (no evidence of congenital vertebra), overall coronal alignment to assess for presence of scoliosis, assess disk height, confirm the presence of two pedicles at each level, and assess soft-tissue shadows, including the psoas muscle. The pelvis and hips should also be evaluated if appropriate, because symptoms often described as back pain may have their origin elsewhere in the general vicinity of the lumbar spine. The lateral radiograph should be assessed for alignment and the presence of normal thoracic kyphosis and lumbar lordosis.[31] Excessive kyphosis in the thoracic region may indicate Scheuermann's kyphosis, congenital kyphosis, osseous spine tumor, or infection. Loss of lordosis in the lumbar spine is often seen with paraspinal muscle contraction associated with significant back pain. Excessive lumbar lordosis can be seen in spondylolisthesis, and the specific subtype should also be identifiable. Detectable radiographic abnormalities include disk space narrowing, vertebral end-plate irregularities, vertebral scalloping, bone lesions, and scoliosis.

It is recommended that further radiographic studies be performed based on each individual patient. If scoliosis is suspected (if the angle of trunk rotation is greater than 7° on scoliometer), 3-foot long cassette standing posteroanterior and lateral radiographs of the thoracolumbar spine are warranted. For spondylolysis, anterior–posterior and lateral plain films of the lumbar spine are often diagnostic. Oblique views can be ordered but may not add significant value in identifying spondylolytic lesions.[32,33] In juvenile onset spondyloarthritis, a single AP view of the pelvis is adequate for the radiographic assessment of the SI joint.[34] Advanced imaging studies should be obtained only after radiographs have been evaluated, since most diagnoses can be made with initial plain radiographs.[6]

Further Workup

Standard three-phase Technetium bone scans are extremely sensitive in identifying a bony abnormality such as an osteoid osteoma or osteoblastoma, but have very low specificity in establishing the diagnosis of spondylolysis. Single-photon emission computed tomography (SPECT) scanning of the lumbar spine is useful and a highly sensitive imaging technique that can accurately localize the pars interarticularis lesion. The advantages of SPECT scans include, (1) ability to diagnose early active lesions before a fracture occurs (i.e. stress reaction or subacute injury to the pars), (2) differentiate between symptomatic and asymptomatic (or silent) pars defects, and (3) determine the chronicity of lesions which may indicate healing potential. Compared to magnetic resonance imaging (MRI), SPECT is less likely to require sedation, can usually be obtained faster at most institutions, and is less expensive. Potential disadvantages of SPECT imaging include the potential for false positives (a hot bone scan on SPECT may be seen in infections, tumors and arthritis), inability to detect a chronic nonunion, and radiation exposure.

A computed tomography (CT) scan is useful for evaluating bony anatomy, and can help localize small bony lesions, such as osteoid osteoma, as well as other bony tumors (such as aneurysmal bone cysts, osteoblastomas), vertebral osteomyelitis, and acute fractures. Three-dimensional reconstructions can be obtained to better represent complex lesions or deformities. CT scans are

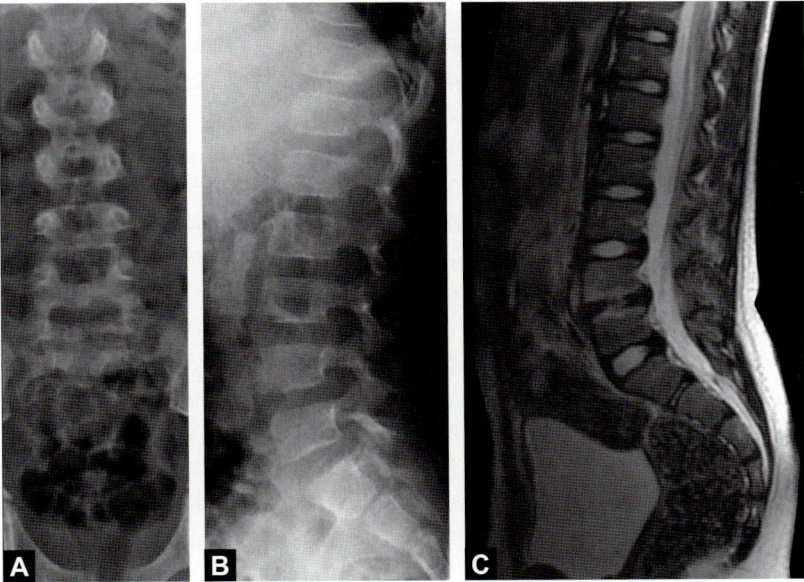

Figs. 1.6A to C: A 6-year-old female with 1-month history of low back pain and limp. (A and B) Initial anteroposterior and lateral radiographs reveal end plate irregularities on the inferior end plate of L4 on the lateral view, (C) Subsequent MRI examination without contrast of the lumbar spine was performed demonstrating findings consistent with both diskitis and vertebral osteomyelitis. A sagittal view T2-Fast Spin Echo weighted image shows loss in L4-5 disk space height, edema within the L4 vertebral body and the superior end plate of L5, and an enhancing fluid collection anterior to the L4 and L5 vertebral bodies.

more specific than SPECT in delineating defects in the pars interarticularis and can help in circumstances when SPECT is positive but nondiagnostic. CT scans can help determine the chronicity of spondylolytic lesions, and are useful as follow-up studies for monitoring healing; however, there is concern for excessive radiation exposure.

Magnetic resonance imaging is excellent at evaluating for intraspinal abnormalities, disk herniations, tumors and infection. Consider obtaining an MRI in the presence of the "red flags" (*see* Box 1.1), or elevated inflammatory indices (erythrocyte sedimentation rate, C-reactive protein), or other concerning symptoms for an infection or malignancy. In diskitis, because plain radiographs may be normal until 3–8 weeks after the onset of symptoms, use of MRI may facilitate early diagnosis, aid recovery, and avoid lengthy hospitalization (Figs. 1.6A to C).[28] In this situation, MRI with gadolinium can differentiate between diskitis, vertebral osteomyelitis, paravertebral inflammation or abscess, and pathology of the hip or spinal cord.[35] MRI is also able to detect and help gauge the chronicity of most spondylolytic lesions, determine the condition of the adjacent intervertebral disks, and exclude canal or foraminal stenosis resulting in neural compression. However, for spondylolytic lesions, MRI has a limited ability to assess cortical integrity to distinguish complete versus incomplete fractures, and to detect bony healing. In adolescent patients, if an apophyseal fracture is suspected on MRI, a CT scan is indicated to evaluate for a slipped vertebral apophysis because it may alter the approach to treatment.[30] With clinical suspicion of spondyloarthritis [back pain for > 3 months, positive human leukocyte antigen B27 (HLA-B27)], MRI may be very helpful to confirm the diagnosis in an early disease stage, providing information on both disease activity and structural damage, without exposing patients to ionizing radiation (a major disadvantage of CT scan).[36]

There are varying opinions and little evidence-based consensus regarding the preferred advanced imaging test to reliably rule out an organic cause of lower back pain in children. Auerbach et al. recommend SPECT imaging in children with non-neurologic back pain of less than 6 weeks duration and MRI for those with persistent pain, particularly with hyperextension testing.[37] If initial radiographs are negative, Feldman et al. recommend MRI in patients with constant pain, night pain, radicular pain, and/or abnormal neurologic examination.[9] Ultimately, the decision to obtain imaging studies in the workup of back pain should be contextual and include diagnostic accuracy, urgency, potential side effects, and limitations of each imaging test.

Laboratory studies, consisting of complete blood count with differential, erythrocyte sedimentation rate, and C-reactive protein should be obtained if there is concern for infection or malignancy (e.g. leukemia). If there is concern for inflammatory arthropathy and spondyloarthritis, HLA-B27 and rheumatoid factor (RF) should be ordered. Lyme disease may sometimes present with diffuse low back pain and is endemic in certain geographical regions.[38] If this condition is suspected, Lyme titers can be tested followed by a Western blot analysis. Urinalysis should also be ordered for flank pain or tenderness, dysuria, or abdominal pain.

CONCLUSION

The prevalence of low back pain in the pediatric population is increasing, but most patients have no specific organic etiology for back pain. The task of evaluating a child with low back pain necessitates a complete understanding of the wide range of disorders that may cause back pain in pediatric patients, and performing a detailed history and physical examination tailored appropriately to the patient's age. Information obtained from the history and clinical examination is critical in identifying children who require symptomatic treatment from those who merit further diagnostic studies. Radiographs of the spine are the best screening examination for the child with back pain and are indicated if the patient is 10 years of age or younger, if there is a history of significant trauma, persistent pain, duration of pain is 2 months or longer, any associated red flags (*see* Box 1.1), or if the clinical findings cannot sufficiently rule out organic causes of back pain. When a serious underlying pathological cause of back pain is suspected, further investigation with diagnostic imaging such as CT scan, MRI, and/or SPECT/ bone scan should be considered on an individual basis.

REFERENCES

1. Olsen TL, Anderson RL, Dearwater SR, et al. The epidemiology of low back pain in an adolescent population. Am J Public Health. 1992;82(4):606-8.
2. Mohseni-Bandpei MA, Bagheri-Nesami M, Shayesteh-Azar M. Nonspecific low back pain in 5000 Iranian school-age children. J Pediatr Orthop. 2007;27(2):126-9.
3. Schmidt CP, Zwingenberger S, Walther A, et al. Prevalence of low back pain in adolescent athletes — an epidemiological investigation. Int J Sports Med. 2014;35(8):684-9.
4. Kujala UM, Taimela S, Erkintalo M, et al. Low-back pain in adolescent athletes. Med Sci Sports Exerc. 1996;28(2):165-70.
5. Iwamoto J, Abe H, Tsukimura Y, et al. Relationship between radiographic abnormalities of lumbar spine and incidence of low back pain in high school and college football players: a prospective study. Am J Sports Med. 2004; 32(3):781-6.
6. Bhatia NN, Chow G, Timon SJ, et al. Diagnostic modalities for the evaluation of pediatric back pain: a prospective study. J Pediatr Orthop. 2008;28(2):230-3.
7. Feldman DS, Hedden DM, Wright JG. The use of bone scan to investigate back pain in children and adolescents. J Pediatr Orthop. 2000;20(6):790-5.
8. Sanpera I, Beguiristain-Gurpide JL. Bone scan as a screening tool in children and adolescents with back pain. J Pediatr Orthop. 2006;26(2):221-5.
9. Feldman DS, Straight JJ, Badra MI, et al. Evaluation of an algorithmic approach to pediatric back pain. J Pediatr Orthop. 2006;26(3):353-7.
10. Balagué F, Nordin M, Skovron ML, et al. Non-specific low-back pain among schoolchildren: a field survey with analysis of some associated factors. J Spinal Disord. 1994;7(5):374-9.
11. Sato T, Ito T, Hirano T, et al. Low back pain in childhood and adolescence: assessment of sports activities. Eur Spine J. 2011;20(1):94-9.
12. Siambanes D, Martinez JW, Butler EW, et al. Influence of school backpacks on adolescent back pain. J Pediatr Orthop. 2004;24(2):211-7.
13. Skoffer B. Low back pain in 15- to 16-year-old children in relation to school furniture and carrying of the school bag. Spine (Phila Pa 1976). 2007;32(24):E713-7.
14. Cardon G, Balagué F. Backpacks and spinal disorders in school children. Eura Medicophys. 2004;40(1):15-20.
15. Skaggs DL, Early SD, D'Ambra P, et al. Back pain and backpacks in school children. J Pediatr Orthop. 2006;26(3):358-63.
16. Gunzburg R, Balagué F, Nordin M, et al. Low back pain in a population of school children. Eur Spine J. 1999;8(6):439-43.
17. Feldman DE, Rossignol M, Shrier I, et al. Smoking. A risk factor for development of low back pain in adolescents. Spine (Phila Pa 1976). 1999;24(23):2492-6.
18. Feldman DE, Shrier I, Rossignol M, et al. Risk factors for the development of low back pain in adolescence. Am J Epidemiol. 2001;154(1):30-6.
19. Turner PG, Green JH, Galasko CS. Back pain in childhood. Spine (Phila Pa 1976). 1989;14(8):812-4.

20. Bono CM. Low-back pain in athletes. J Bone Joint Surg Am. 2004;86-A(2): 382-96.
21. Quinlan JF, Duke D, Eustace S. Bertolotti's syndrome. A cause of back pain in young people. J Bone Joint Surg Br. 2006;88(9):1183-6.
22. Mangla J, Young JL, Young JO, et al. Sacral stress fractures in children. Am J Orthop (Belle Mead NJ). 2009;38(5):232-6.
23. Rabb CH, McComb JG, Raffel C, et al. Spinal arachnoid cysts in the pediatric age group: an association with neural tube defects. J Neurosurg. 1992;77(3): 369-72.
24. Lipton G, Riddle E, Grissom L, et al. An unusual cause of low-back pain in children: a report of two cases. J Bone Joint Surg Am. 2001;83-A(10):1552-4.
25. Hershkovich O, Friedlander A, Gordon B, et al. Associations of body mass index and body height with low back pain in 829,791 adolescents. Am J Epidemiol. 2013;178(4):603-9.
26. Samartzis D, Karppinen J, Mok F, et al. A population-based study of juvenile disc degeneration and its association with overweight and obesity, low back pain, and diminished functional status. J Bone Joint Surg Am. 2011;93(7): 662-70.
27. Phalen GS, Dickson JA. Spondylolisthesis and tight hamstrings. J Bone Joint Surg Am. 1961(43-A):505-12.
28. Brown R, Hussain M, McHugh K, et al. Discitis in young children. J Bone Joint Surg Br. 2001;83(1):106-11.
29. Katz K, Rosenthal A, Yosipovitch Z. Normal ranges of popliteal angle in children. J Pediatr Orthop. 1992;12(2):229-31.
30. Frino J, McCarthy RE, Sparks CY, et al. Trends in adolescent lumbar disk herniation. J Pediatr Orthop. 2006;26(5):579-81.
31. Mac-Thiong JM, Berthonnaud E, Dimar JR, et al. Sagittal alignment of the spine and pelvis during growth. Spine (Phila Pa 1976). 2004;29(15):1642-7.
32. Miller R, Beck NA, Sampson NR, et al. Imaging modalities for low back pain in children: a review of spondyloysis and undiagnosed mechanical back pain. J Pediatr Orthop. 2013;33(3):282-8.
33. Beck NA, Miller R, Baldwin K, et al. Do oblique views add value in the diagnosis of spondylolysis in adolescents? J Bone Joint Surg Am. 2013;95(10):e65.
34. Maksymowych WP. Controversies in conventional radiography in spondyloarthritis. Best Pract Res Clin Rheumatol. 2012;26(6):839-52.
35. Du Lac P, Panuel M, Devred P, et al. MRI of disc space infection in infants and children. Report of 12 cases. Pediatr Radiol. 1990;20(3):175-8.
36. Pedersen SJ, Weber U, Ostergaard M. The diagnostic utility of MRI in spondyloarthritis. Best Pract Res Clin Rheumatol. 2012;26(6):751-66.
37. Auerbach JD, Ahn J, Zgonis MH, et al. Streamlining the evaluation of low back pain in children. Clin Orthop Relat Res. 2008;466(8):1971-7.
38. Kameda G, Vieker S, Hartmann J, et al. Diastolic heart murmur, nocturnal back pain, and lumbar rigidity in a 7-year girl: an unusual manifestation of lyme disease in childhood. Case Rep Pediatr. 2012;2012:976961.

CHAPTER 2

Lower Back Pain in Adults

Tim Colangelo, John D Koerner, Alexander R Vaccaro

INTRODUCTION

Low back pain is a very common complaint among adults. A typical case scenario may be as follows: a 50-year-old male reports low lumbar back pain of 1 year duration. He experiences pain and stiffness that is exasperated by standing for long periods of time and upon rising from a sitting position. He describes a persistent pain in the middle of his lower back that has intensified over the last few weeks. Patient reports progressively worsening of symptoms that have begun to interfere with normal daily activities. Patient states mild relief from over-the-counter analgesic. There was no previous trauma or identifiable incident.

DIFFERENTIAL DIAGNOSIS

Low back pain is an unfortunate common complaint and due to the wide array of manifestations it can make forming a differential diagnosis an arduous task. In arriving at a conclusion, the patient's age, location/quality of pain, presenting symptoms, thorough history and physical exam, as well as imaging studies will lead to optimal workup and subsequent diagnosis. Here we briefly outline possible diagnoses based on the patient's chief complaint and history beginning with the more common causes and ending with rare conditions (Box 2.1).

ANATOMY

A detailed understanding of the anatomy of the lower spine and associated structures is imperative in the correct diagnosis for a patient presenting with low back pain. The low back starts at the lumbar vertebra L1 and extends through the 5 fused sacral vertebrae and 3–4 coccygeal vertebrae. The posterior spinous processes of the 5 lumbar vertebrae are usually palpable through the skin. The ligamentum flavum attaches to the laminae of adjacent

Box 2.1: Differential diagnoses for low back pain.
• Muscular strain/sprain
• Degenerative disk disease
• Herniated disk
• Osteoporosis and compression fractures
• Lumbar spinal stenosis
• Degenerative scoliosis
• Cauda equina syndrome
• Spondylolisthesis
• Ankylosing spondylitis
• Non-mechanical spinal condition and visceral disease

vertebrae from C2 to the sacrum. The ligament provides support and preserves the upright posture. The paravertebral muscles also provide added support and mobility to the axial skeleton.

Fibrocartilaginous intervertebral disks are positioned between vertebrae. They are composed of an outer annulus fibrosus and an inner nucleus pulposus. The disks serve as shock absorbers and provide protection and flexibility between stacked vertebrae. These disks progressively deteriorate and flatten with age. In the case of a patient with degenerative disk disease, this deterioration is accelerated and leads to pain emanating from the disk and often leads to a disk rupture or herniation. With herniation, the inner nucleus pulposus can protrude into the canal or foramen causing neural compression (Fig. 2.1).

Anterior and posterior longitudinal ligaments line the vertebral column (Fig. 2.2). The posterior ligament is weaker and less developed, especially at the lateral edges. Disk herniation, therefore, most often occurs in the posterolateral direction and impinges on the spinal nerves in the vertebral foramina causing associated symptoms (Fig. 2.1). Herniated disks occur most frequently at levels L3-L4, L4-L5, and L5-S1, and involve the L4, L5, and S1 nerve roots. The spinal nerve roots pass through their respected intervertebral foramen immediately lateral to the associated intervertebral disk. In the lumbar spine, a herniated disk can compress the lower emerging root and produce pain and numbness in the associated dermatome.

The cauda equina may be compressed with a massive midline disk herniation, spinal stenosis, infection, inflammatory disease, or space occupying lesions causing cauda equina syndrome. The cauda equina is composed of dorsal and ventral roots of the lower lumbar and sacral nerves (L1-S5). They begin at the conus medullaris usually opposite the disk between L1 and L2 and the lower spinal nerve roots must travel within the lumbar cistern to reach their respective intervertebral foramina.

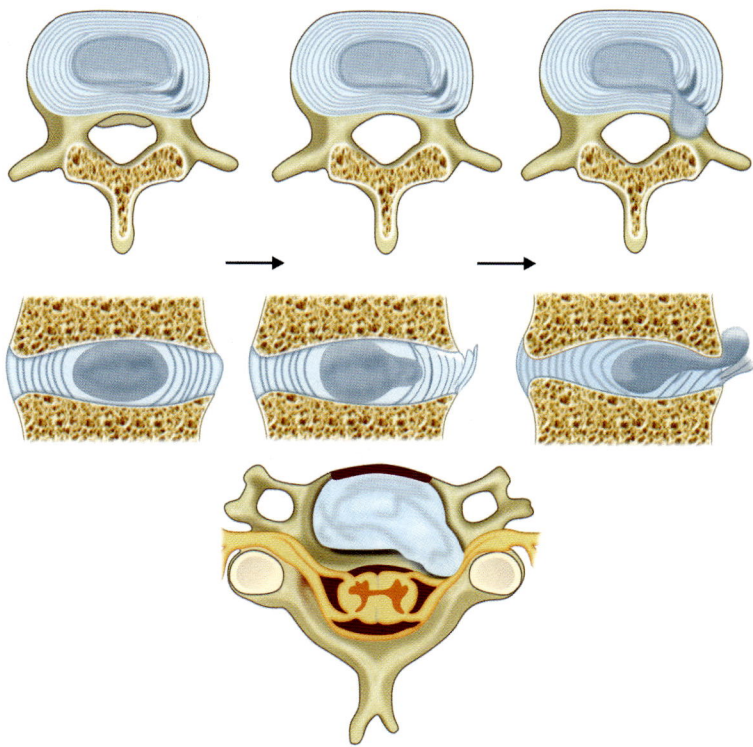

Fig. 2.1: Progression of a disk herniation with the inner nucleus pulposus protruding into the neural foramen.

Vertebral ligaments

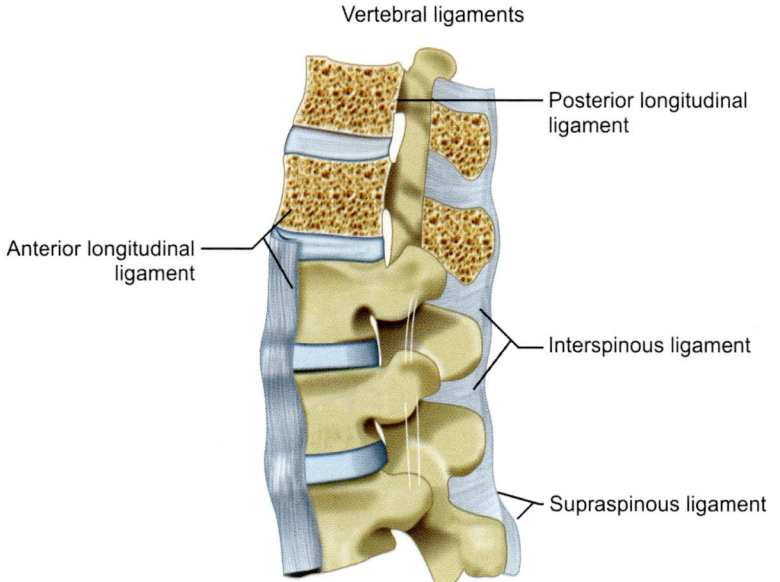

Posterior longitudinal ligament

Anterior longitudinal ligament

Interspinous ligament

Supraspinous ligament

Fig. 2.2: Anatomy of the lumbar spine.

PHYSICAL EXAM

The goal in the evaluation of patients with low back pain is to ascertain the source of the pain and to identify patients who have a serious underlying disorder from those with a less urgent mechanical stress related discomfort, i.e. muscle strain (Table 2.1).

Identifying the contributing structures for patients presenting with low back pain is difficult as multiple structures are often involved. Clinicians should focus on provocative factors, quality of pain, location, radiation, severity, and timing. Clinical assessment should define the degree of pain, functional limitations, range of motion, and other possible contributing factors. The physical examination should assess posture to identify any skeletal irregularities or deformities. The spine and lower extremities should be thoroughly examined. The site of pain or tenderness should be noted as well as any signs of gait abnormalities or restriction of movement. The clinician must be cognizant of other involved systems as the pain may be referred.

Table 2.1: Etiology and features of low back pain.[1]

Possible cause	Key features on history/exam
Herniated disk	• Back and leg pain in an L4, L5 or S1 nerve pathway • Positive straight leg test or crossed straight leg test
Spinal stenosis	• Radiating leg pain • Older age • Reduced lumbar extension • Improvement in pain with lumbar flexion
Vertebral compression fracture	• History of osteoporosis • Use of corticosteroids • Postmenopausal woman
Degenerative scoliosis	• Lateral deviation of spine • Axial back pain • Neurogenic claudication • Older age (> 50 years old)
Cauda equina syndrome	• Urinary retention • Fecal incontinence • Saddle anesthesia • Sexual dysfunction
Ankylosing spondylitis	• Morning stiffness • Awakening in middle of night due to back pain • Improvement with exercise • Younger age
Cancer	• History of cancer • Unexplained weight loss • Pain that does not subside with rest

In many cases, low back pain results from non-specific mechanical and postural stresses on the spine. Straining of the muscles that support the vertebral column will cause discomfort. The patient will present with local tenderness and limited range of motion. The pain is most often described as an ache and the patient may experience back spasms. The pain is exasperated by physical activity, bending, and changing position. This diagnosis is atypical if the patient presents with associated neurogenic claudication or radiculopathy.

Posture can be indicative of many spinal disorders. The shoulders and pelvis should be level and there should be bilateral symmetry. There should be a normal lordotic curvature of the lumbar spine and any deviations from this should be noted. Any disease that weakens or degenerates the vertebrae will often cause patients to present with compensatory kyphosis.

Compensatory kyphosis is found in patients with lumbar spinal stenosis. The differential diagnosis of lumbar spinal stenosis is expansive due to the various and frequent coexistence of other spinal pathologies. Any pathology that causes a narrowing of the spinal canal space can lead to spinal stenosis. Reduced and painful lumbar extension that is relieved with lumbar flexion is a clinically significant finding in patients with lumbar spinal stenosis.[6] Forward flexed gait may also be present.

Patients with osteoporosis may also present with compensatory kyphosis. The disease is most commonly found in older, thin, postmenopausal women; however, it can affect males as well. Osteoporosis predisposes the patient to compression fractures in the spine and can be a source of pain. A lumbar vertebral compression fracture may be present when an older patient presents with low back pain of acute onset with or without specific history of recent injury. While not sufficient alone, the physical exam is important in the diagnosis of osteoporosis and should include a thorough evaluation of the patient. Later in the chapters, we will discuss additional laboratory workup that will help in arriving at a diagnosis for osteoporosis.

It is important to ascertain discogenic back pain from nondiscogenic pain. Discogenic pain is often described occurring in the midline of the low back. The pathology will be within the intervertebral disks. Sustained hip flexion will increase pressure within the intervertebral disk. Reproducible midline low back pain in this position with movement of the pelvis has been shown to be predictive of discogenic pathology in patients under the age of 55 years old.[14] The Centralization Phenomenon described by McKenzie, is another method for differentiating between discogenic and nondiscogenic pain.[15] The technique uses end-range lumbar movements to progressively move pain away from distal extremities toward the proximal lumbar midline. Therefore centralization occurs when pain moves from its most distal position toward the lumbar midline and a positive test may be indicative of discogenic-related pathology.

In degenerative disk disease, the intervertebral disks supporting the vertebrae degrade at a pathological rate. Prolonged standing and flexion may exasperate the pain. Most patients will find relief with extension. As the dehydrated disk is compressed between the vertebrae it is possible for the nucleus pulposus to break through or rupture the outer annulus fibrosus. This leads to the finding of disk herniation and is often associated with progressive degenerative disk disease.

Degenerative scoliosis or "de novo" scoliosis is another relatively common cause of low back pain predominating in patients older than 50 years of age. This postural deformity is associated with a previously straight spine distinguishing it from adult scoliosis. It is characterized by asymmetrical degeneration of the intervertebral disks and facet joints often leading to neurologic claudication with associated radicular leg pain. The most common findings include lateral listhesis, loss of lumbar lordosis, axial back pain, and spinal imbalance.[17] Patients may present with extreme lower back pain and lower extremity pain. Rarely, coronal or sagittal imbalance may be apparent. Physical exam should seek to evaluate the source of pain and will include a neurological exam of the extremities. Hyperextension of the lumbar spine may exacerbate the pain in either the lower back or lower extremities. The clinician should assess leg length discrepancies, rib impingement, lumbar flexibility, spinal alignment and any loss of height.[17] Further diagnostic imaging tests will confirm a diagnosis.

A thorough palpation of the lumbar spine will aid in identifying any irregularities within each vertebra. A palpable step-off from one spinous process to another may be indicative of spondylolisthesis. First, locate the superior aspect of the iliac crest. Placing your thumbs on the midline of the back will often put you directly at the L4-L5 interspace. This can be used as a reference point for identifying the rest of vertebrae.

Spondylolisthesis is caused by the slippage of a vertebra anteriorly out of its physiological position. There are a number of different types of spondylolisthesis. The most common to present in the adult include degenerative and spondylolytic spondylolisthesis. Degenerative spondylolisthesis is due mostly to degeneration of the components of the spinal unit over time. Degeneration of the intervertebral disks and the development of facet osteoarthritis weaken the joints and put an increasing amount of pressure on the ligamentum flavum, which holds the vertebrae in their proper position. When a vertebra overcomes this resistance, it will slip compressing the spinal canal and cause pain. The patient usually experiences general stiffening and pain in the lower back at the site of the slip. Prolonged standing and walking aggravate the pain. Neurogenic claudication may be found.

Spondylolytic spondylolisthesis is due to a fracture in the pars interarticularis. The pars interarticularis fracture causes the vertebrae and the lamina to disconnect and thus only the front of the vertebra slips forward.

This makes it less likely to cause a narrowing of the spinal canal as seen in degenerative spondylolisthesis. Patients with this manifestation are less likely to present with symptoms typical of lumbar stenosis and neurological deficits are seldom found.

The exam should include a detailed assessment of neurological function. Neurological tests are imperative in order to determine if nerve roots are irritated. The lower extremities are examined as lower spinal nerve pathologies often manifest in these extremities in the form of altered reflexes, loss of cutaneous sensation, and decreased muscle strength. The examination should be conducted along neurological lines following the path of the spinal nerves. At each spinal level reflexes, sensation and muscle strength will be evaluated.

A number of tests are available to stretch nerve roots. The sciatic nerve can be palpated as well. To palpate the sciatic nerve, have the patient flex his hip, locate the midpoint between the ischial tuberosity and greater trochanter and firmly press at the midpoint. Furthermore, a straight-leg raise test should be performed in patients with possible nerve root dysfunction. The test may indicate the presence of a herniated disk in the lumbar spine and will help in making decisions regarding diagnostic imaging. It is possible for the intervertebral disks to weaken and bulge or herniate out of the physiological joint space. This can be caused by trauma, but is most often secondary to degeneration of the disks. This should be suspected when the patient presents with sharp shooting pain and associated paresthesia in the leg or buttocks. The pain is often described as continuous and can be relieved or worsened by changing position depending on where the herniation has occurred.

If herniated disk is suspected the level and extent must be clarified. Central midline disk herniation may compress the nerve roots of the cauda equina leading to cauda equina syndrome. Urinary retention is the most common finding associated with cauda equina syndrome. Loss of bowel control and sexual dysfunction are other common findings. Motor weakness, and sensory loss around the thigh and buttocks (saddle anesthesia) may also be present in this condition.

To perform the straight-leg raise test, have the patient lay in the supine position and lift the leg upward and support the foot around the heel. If this maneuver produces a painful reaction, lower the leg slightly from the level at which the patient first experiences the pain and dorsiflex the foot to stretch the sciatic nerve (Fig. 2.3). A positive reaction from dorsiflexion could be confirmative of pathology. Follow up this test with the straight-leg raise test on the well leg (contralateral straight-leg raise test). With the patient still supine raise the uninvolved leg (Fig. 2.4). If this produces pain on the opposite side this is further evidence that indicates irritation to the nerve.

The physician should also be alert to other rare causes of low back pain during the physical exam. Ankylosing spondylitis (AS) is an autoimmune

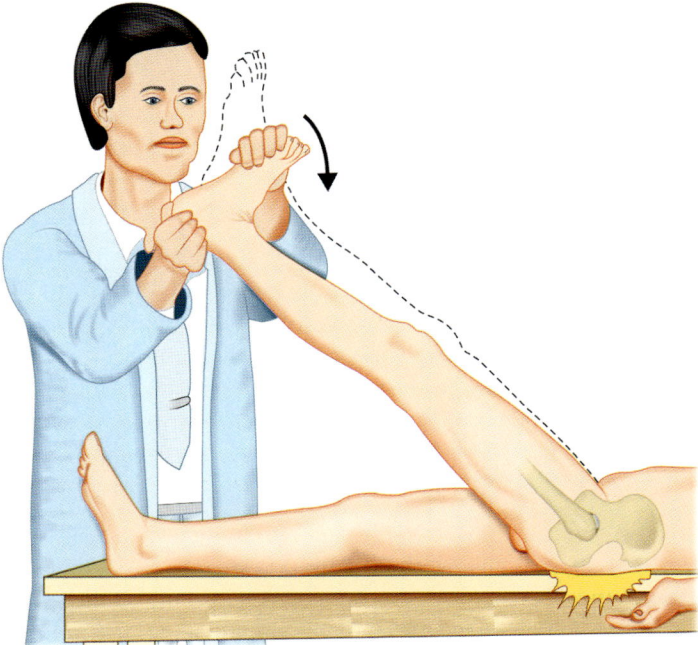

Fig. 2.3: Straight leg raising test with dorsiflexion.[4]

inflammatory disease of the vertebral joints most often presenting in adult males. It is considered a type III hypersensitivity and results in the deposition of immune complexes in the vertebral joints. The patient will present with back pain and stiffness particularly in the morning hours upon awakening. The disease eventually will result in damage to the joints, fusion of the sacroiliac joints (sacroiliitis) and ankylosing of the vertebrae. The patient will usually describe the pain as progressive over weeks or months rather than days. Osteitis, ossification within the annulus fibrosus, and erosions are the vertebral manifestations of AS.[9]

Rarely, low back pain is caused by non-mechanical conditions or visceral disease, i.e. neoplasm or an abdominal aortic aneurysm. Metastatic cancer may also cause low back pain. A history of previous cancer, unexplained weight loss, and pain that does not subside with rest all could be indicative of a cancerous etiology. Any malignant growths around the spine can impinge upon the spinal cord and nerve roots. These growths may be palpable upon physical examination. Patients with an early abdominal aortic aneurysm will often be asymptomatic. Pain will develop and radiate to the back as the aneurysm enlarges. The aneurysm may be found on physical exam.

It is also important to consider the possibility of social factors contributing to the patient's complaints. Psychological issues such as stress and depression may be associated with the progression of acute to chronic low back pain.[15]

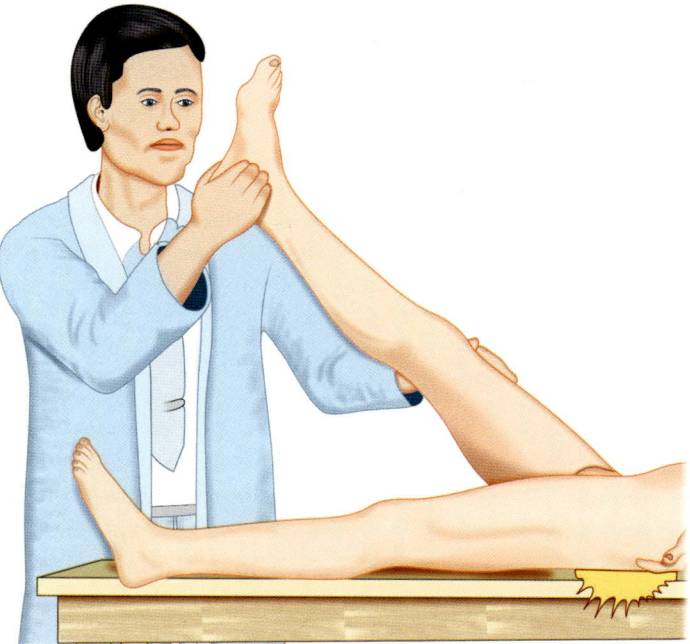

Fig. 2.4: Positive cross leg straight-leg raising test.

IMAGING STUDIES

Imaging tests are necessary when patients present with symptoms in the physical exam that suggest progressive neurologic deficit or a severe underlying disorder. Imaging studies should be obtained only to confirm a diagnosis based on history and physical exam.

In suspected degenerative disk disease, plain radiographs are the first approach at evaluation.[5] They will help to rule out pain caused by fracture, deformity, or metastasis; however, follow up with more sensitive computed tomography (CT) or magnetic resonance imaging (MRI) is often necessary to make a definitive diagnosis. Telling findings upon MRI includes disk space narrowing, loss of T2 signal within nucleus pulposus, end plate changes, and signs of disk tear.[5] Pfirrmann et al. developed a grading system for the assessment of lumbar disk degeneration using T-2 weighted MRI sequences.[3] The morphologic grading system is based on a scale of I–V and analyzes the degree of disk degeneration. Grade I disks are white, homogeneous with a clear distinction between nucleus and annulus and a normal disk space height (Fig. 2.5A). Grade II disks are heterogeneous with banding, clear distinction between nucleus and annulus and normal disk space height (Fig. 2.5B). Grade III disks are gray with unclear distinction between nucleus and annulus and a normal to decreased disk space height (Fig. 2.5C).

Grade IV disks are gray to black with no distinction between nucleus and annulus and a normal to decreased disk space height (Fig. 2.5D). Grade V disks are black and show a true collapsed disk space (Fig. 2.5E). This grading system provides a standardized assessment of MRI classification of disk degeneration.

Plain radiographs are valuable in assessing disk height, but not capable of diagnosing disk tear or herniation. MRI is the preferred diagnostic imaging procedure for patients with suspected disk herniation. The extent of disk herniation morphology is classified into: normal, bulge, and herniation (protrusion or extrusion as subcategories). A bulge is defined as a symmetrical invasion of the disk outside of the normal joint space. Disk herniation is an asymmetrical invasion of the disk outside of the normal joint space. Herniations can be subdivided into extrusions or protrusions based upon their shape (Figs. 2.6A and B). An extrusion is described as a base that is narrower than the extruded part of the disk while a protrusion has a broader base.[8,9] Bulges and protrusions are more commonly found in asymptomatic individuals.[9]

Plain film radiography should be the first approach in patients with suspected degenerative scoliosis. These will show the extent of deformity, curve location, and number of levels. The Cobb method should be utilized to measure the coronal angle of the curvature on the standing anteroposterior (AP) radiograph. Sagittal alignment is measured on the full length lateral radiographs by drawing a plumb line from the C7 vertebral body and measuring the distance to the posterior L5/S1 disk space. MRI, CT scan, and myelography can provide additional information regarding neural, soft tissue, and vertebral anatomy.

In patients with suspected lumbar spinal stenosis MRI has the highest sensitivity and is the preferred method to confirm a diagnosis, as plain film radiography cannot accurately assess the degree of stenosis.[7] The clinician will rate a patient with mild, moderate, or severe lumbar spinal stenosis. The general guideline for classifying the patient is the extent of narrowing of the normal central canal cross-sectional area. Mild stenosis classifies as a narrowing of one-third its normal size, moderate stenosis is a narrowing between one-third and two thirds, and severe stenosis is a compromise of greater than two-thirds its normal size.[2,7]

Plain film radiograph can identify vertebral compression fractures when they are clearly defined. However, MRI may be necessary in the absence of obvious deformity, as is the case with non-displaced stress fractures.[11] MRI is also useful in differentiating between acute and chronic fractures. CT scan can be used to rule out unstable spinal fractures.

A dual-energy X-ray absorptiometry (DXA) scan measures bone mineral density and is used to identify those who either have osteoporosis or at risk of developing osteoporosis. The World Health Organization has developed guidelines in the classification of osteoporosis through the DXA

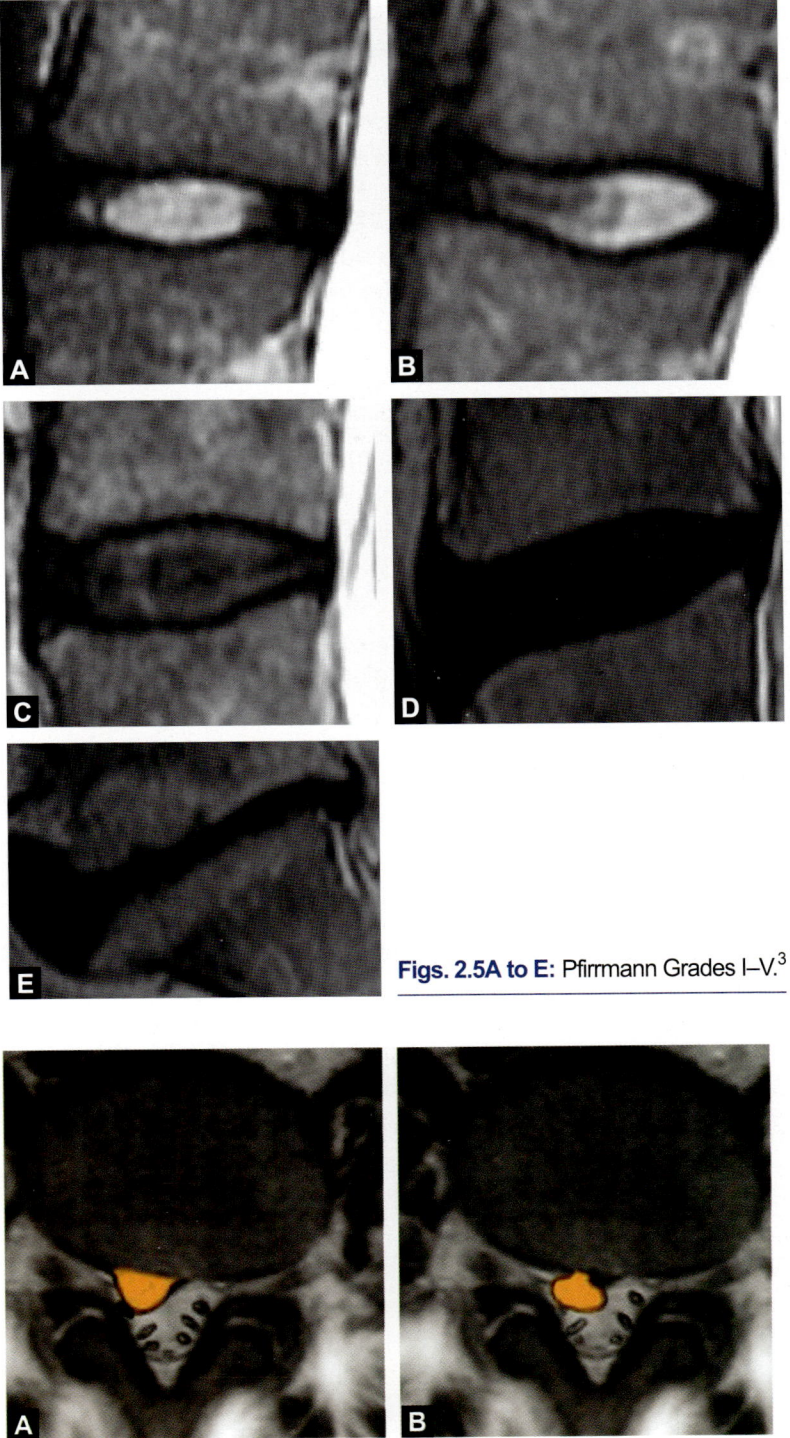

Figs. 2.5A to E: Pfirrmann Grades I–V.[3]

Figs. 2.6A and B: Protrusion (A) versus extrusion (B).[16]

scan. A T-score between –1 and –2.5 is considered osteopenia or mild bone deficiency. A T-score of less than or equal to –2.5 is indicative of a diagnosis of osteoporosis. Patients with previous fragility fractures and a T-score less than –2.5 indicate severe osteoporosis. End plate vertebral fractures are a common consequence of increased fragility in the osteoporotic spine.

Plain radiograph is sufficient to visualize the bony changes and to identify spondylolisthesis. MRI or CT scan will provide a more detailed picture including soft tissue disruption and is necessary when the patient is experiencing neurologic deficits, as this will allow identification of the affected nerves.

FURTHER WORKUP

Further workup will aid in arriving at a concluisive diagnosis. Certain markers can be a clear indicator of causes of low back pain and thus laboratory tests are a useful tool in forming a differential diagnosis.

Osteoporosis

In patients with a suspected osteoporotic compression fracture, initial laboratory tests should include those tests identifying specific bone markers. These would include vitamin D levels, serum calcium, phosphate, alkaline phosphatase, and magnesium. In order to ascertain possible secondary causes, thyroid stimulating hormone, 24-hour urine calcium, and parathyroid hormone level should be evaluated.

Ankylosing Spondylitis

Ankylosing spondylitis can be confirmed using imaging tests in conjunction with laboratory markers. A blood test should be conducted to check for the presence of the human leukocyte antigen (HLA)-B27 antigen. HLA-B27 is a class I major histocompatibility complex that is involved in the progression of AS. Having the gene does not necessarily translate to disease, but can aid in a correct diagnosis.

Plain film radiograph can identify sacroiliitis, an early and common finding in AS. MRI can identify acute inflammation. The finding of sacroiliitis with the presence of one or more features of axial spondyloarthritis is confirmative of the pathology. The Assessment of SpondyloArthritis International Society published literature defining consensus classification of AS which includes patients with back pain onset before 45 years of age and with more than 3 months of pain:[10]

- Sacroiliitis on imaging plus one or more features of axial spondyloarthritis or;
- +HLA-B27 plus two or more features of axial spondyloarthritis.

A myelogram is an alternative radiographic imaging technique that takes advantage of contrast media dyes to visualize the spinal cord and associated pathology. It can be used on patients who are unable to undergo MRI and can aid in detecting the source of pain.

Finally, diskography is a technique used in evaluating discogenic low back pain. It can specify which specific disks are causing the patient pain when all other diagnostic tests have failed. Due to the large instances of false positives and the potential to cause iatrogenic disk injury this test has been met with rising controversy over recent years.[13] However, the power of this test is the fact that seemingly normal disk anatomically may be generating pain due to internal disruption, i.e. annular fissure. Injecting contrast media into the disks pressurizes the space inducing pain. The standard criteria of a positive result on diskogram are as follows: (1) injection must produce significant pain; (2) the pain must be similar to the patient's normal pain and (3) a control disk must produce no pain.[12] The ability for patients to distinguish discogenic pain from other sources is also questionable, therefore results should be interpreted with caution and patients to undergo diskography should be carefully selected.

CONCLUSION

Low back pain in adults is a troubling clinical presentation for a physician due to the extreme variability in symptoms and the number of various etiologies. This emphasizes the importance of forming a concrete and focused differential diagnosis. It is imperative to conduct a thorough history and physical exam before moving on to more detailed imaging techniques and workup. Low back pain imparts a large socioeconomic toll on the health care system and the prevalence will continue to rise as the population ages.

REFERENCES

1. Chou R, Qaseem A, Snow V, et al. Diagnosis and treatment of low back pain: a joint clinical practice guideline from the American College of Physicians and the American Pain Society. Ann Intern Med. 2007;147(7):478-91.
2. Suri P, Rainville J, Kalichman L, et al. Does this older adult with lower extremity pain have the clinical syndrome of lumbar spinal stenosis? JAMA. 2010;304(23):2628-36.
3. Pfirrmann CW, Metzdorf A, Zanetti M, et al. Magnetic resonance classification of lumbar intervertebral disc degeneration. Spine. 2001;26(17):1873-8.
4. Hoppenfeld S, Hutton R (Eds). Physical Examination of the Spine and Extremities. Upper Saddle River, NJ: Prentice Hall; 1976.
5. Taher F, Essig D, Lebl DR, et al. Lumbar degenerative disc disease: current and future concepts of diagnosis and management. Adv Orthop. 2012;970752.
6. Katz JN, Harris MB. Clinical practice: lumbar spinal stenosis. N Engl J Med. 2008;358(8):818-25.

7. de Schepper El, Overdevest GM, Suri P, et al. Diagnosis of lumbar spinal stenosis: an updated systematic review of the accuracy of diagnostic tests. Spine. 2013;38(8):E469-81.

8. Fardon DF, Milette PC. Nomenclature and classification of lumbar disc pathology. Recommendations of the Combined task Forces of the North American Spine Society, American Society of Spine Radiology, and American Society of Neuroradiology. Spine. 2001;26(5):E93-E113.

9. Jarvik JG, Deyo RA. Diagnostic evaluation of low back pain with emphasis on imaging. Ann Intern Med. 2002;37(7):586-97.

10. Rudwaleit M, van der Heijde D, Landewé R, et al. The development of Assessment of SpondyloArthritis International Society classification criteria for axial spondyloarthritis (part II): validation and final selection. Ann Rheum Dis. 2009;68(6):777-83.

11. Kim DH, Vaccaro AR. Osteoporotic compression fractures of the spine; current options and considerations for treatment. Spine. 2006; 6(5):479-87.

12. Walsh TR, Weinstein JN, Spratt KF, et al. Lumbar discography in normal subjects. A controlled, prospective study. J Bone Joint Surg Am. 1990;72(7):1081-8.

13. Carragee EJ, Chen Y, Tanner CM, et al. Can discography cause long-term back symptoms in previously asymptomatic subjects? Spine. 2000;25(14):1803-8.

14. DePalma MK J, Queler E, Ruchala M, et al. Multivariate analysis of predictor variables of low back pain: an interim analysis of a cross sectional analytic study. The Spine Journal: official journal of the North American Spine Society. 2009;9(10S):143S.

15. Pincus T, Burton AK, Vogel S, et al. A systematic review of psychological factors as predictors of chronicity/disability in prospective cohorts of low back pain. Spine. 2002;27(5):E109-20.

16. The Radiology Assistant. (2014). The Educational site of the Radiological Society of the Netherlands. [internet] Available from http://www.radiologyassistant.nl. [Accessed July, 2015].

17. Tribus CB. Degenerative lumbar scoliosis: evaluation and management. J Am Acad Orthop Surg. 2003;11(3):174-83.

CHAPTER 3

Arm Pain, Weakness and Numbness

Angela Chang, Caleb Behrend, Alexander R Vaccaro

INTRODUCTION

Musculoskeletal injuries and overuse of joints are the most common causes of upper limb pain and weakness. Pain, sensory disturbances and weakness are associated with neural compression and may be readily apparent upon physical examination with repetitive motion. It is important to identify the source of patient symptoms as well as associated symptoms as damage to upper and lower motor tracts may be the diagnoses. Narrowing of anatomical locations may contribute to discomfort and vascular constriction, and signs of cyanosis or insufficient vascular supply to peripheral tissues may be readily apparent upon visual inspection. Nerve conduction tests and electromyography (EMG), imaging studies and lab workup may be appropriate to confirm diagnosis.

CHIEF COMPLAINT/HISTORY

Patient may notice or complain of generalized neck and arm pain or weakness with a tingling sensation in the forearm and fingers upon evaluation. When taking the history, have the patient elaborate upon their symptoms. Ask the patient about the onset of symptoms, quality of the pain (continuous, intermittent, or throbbing), specific location, severity, frequency, radiation, associated symptoms, if there have been previous similar experiences and what actions alleviate or exacerbate symptoms. The past medical history should include any prior trauma, infections (may provide indications of acute or chronic infections), neurological symptoms, surgical procedures and relevant family history. It may be important for the clinician to ask about previous diagnosis of diabetes, immune suppression or cancer. The clinician should observe patient's gait and note any limitations, including discomfort or compensatory mechanisms, of range of movement at neck, shoulder, upper limb joints and spine. Symptoms such as sensory deficit, fevers, chills or unexplained weight loss should be noted. Bulbar symptoms such as

Box 3.1: Upper limb pain and weakness history: pertinent red flags.
• Trauma
• Unexplained significant motor and/or sensory loss (indications of neurological lesions)
• Lesions, tenderness or swelling (indications of tumor or infections)
• History of cancer
• Persistent or progressive pain that is unresponsive to NSAIDs
• Pain at rest, including night pain

(NSAIDs: Nonsteroidal anti-inflammatory drugs).

difficulty in swallowing food and liquids, facial weakness, or excess salivation may be indicative of progressive weakness or degeneration of motor neurons extending above the spinal cord.

Motor and sensory abnormalities need to be carefully assessed by the clinician. If the patient has spinal cord injury, it must be recognized and treated early to reduce the possibility of permanent loss of function. Physical examination of the spine and upper limb should include palpations for bony abnormalities, noting any tenderness, areas of redness, blisters or other irregularities. Such findings are red flag indicators (Box 3.1).

If patient describes a pattern of pain consistent with cardiac origin including uncomfortable tightness of chest and radiation from chest to the arm (neck and jaw), shortness of breath and lightheadedness, seek immediate emergency care.

DIFFERENTIAL DIAGNOSIS

An extensive range of pathologies can result in upper limb pain and/or weakness (Table 3.1). Though causes of upper limb pain or weakness are primarily attributed to the overuse of muscles and joints, loss of neuronal integrity (compression and/or degeneration) can produce similar symptoms along with sensory deficits. Progressive muscle weakness or muscular strength throughout the day may be indicative of an autoimmune disease. Progressive and chronic muscular weakness may be reflective of central nervous system (CNS) pathology. Management of symptoms should begin with non-invasive therapies such as injections of local anesthetic and prescription of nonsteroidal anti-inflammatory drugs (NSAIDs) to provide relief and muscle strengthening with physical or occupational therapy, prior to consideration of surgical intervention.

ANATOMY/PHYSICAL EXAM

Prior to physical exam, evaluation of patient history should include the patient's ability to carry out daily routines and activities. Recall key elements

Table 3.1: Differential diagnosis of common spinal causes of upper limb pain/weakness.[7, 16-20, 24, 25]

	Presenting characteristics of upper limb pain	Associated symptoms
Muscular strain	• Sudden onset of pain • Soreness • Limited range of motion	• Bruising or discoloration • Swelling • Muscle spasms • Stiffness • Weakness
Compressive neuropathy	• Signs of thoracic outlet syndrome of neurogenic origin • Signs of carpal tunnel syndrome	• Sensory deficit
Tendonitis	• Pain or tenderness at joint	• Swelling • Stiffness
Rotator cuff tear	• Pain at rest and during motion • Weakness	• Crepitus
SLAP tear	• Crepitus, popping or clicking with motion • Pain • Weakness	• Sense of instability at shoulder joint • Ache
Cervical radiculopathy	• Sharp pain that extends to periphery	• Pins and needles sensation • Weakness
Cervical myelopathy	• Upper limb pain • Tingling • Muscle weakness	• Irregular movements • Lightheadedness • Problem with fine motor movements
Angina or myocardial infarction	• Pain and squeezing sensation of chest • Pain radiation to left shoulder	• Jaw pain (pain extension to the neck) • Sweating • Nausea • Belching (more prevalent in females) • No symptoms
Thoracic outlet syndrome	• Pain in neck, shoulder or hand • Tingling or numbness down the arm	• Cramping upon repetitive activity (sign of claudication) • Muscle wasting
Malignancy (compression of spinal or peripheral nerves)	• Radiating pain • Numbness or tingling	• Muscle weakness
Spinal infection	• Fever • Chills • Pain	• Tenderness • Stiffness • Erythema

Contd…

Contd…

	Presenting characteristics of upper limb pain	Associated symptoms
Fracture	• Abnormal contour • Pain • Swelling or bruising	• Loss of function
Fibromyalgia	• Generalize muscular or joint pain • Depression • Fatigue • Anxiety	• Concentration and memory problems • Headaches • Irritable bowel syndrome • Morning stiffness • Sleeping problems • Numbness and tingling of upper limb
Cerebrovascular event	• Sudden unilateral numbness or weakness of face and arm • Confusion	• Blurred vision • Loss of balance
Radial head dislocation (Pediatric)	• Pain • Hanging arm • Disuse of arm	• No swelling or deformity
Erb-Duchenne palsy	• Discomfort of shoulder • Stiff and crooked appearance of arm	• Circulatory problems and associated cramps
Amyotrophic lateral sclerosis	• Progressive muscle weakness, cramping, fasciculations and spasticity	• Abnormal fatigue • Slurred speech • Respiratory failure
Compartment syndrome	• Intense pain, worse with motion • Paresthesia	• Numbness or paralysis • Difficulty moving • Muscle bulging
Syringomyelia	• Loss of hot/cold sensitivity • Numbness and tingling • Muscle weakness • Pain	• Paralysis • Bowl and bladder dysfunction
Multiple sclerosis	• Numbness or weakness of limb • Loss of vision • Loss of coordination of muscles	• Dysarthria and dysphagia • Muscle spasm • Bowel and bladder dysfunction
Myasthenia gravis	• Progressive weakness throughout the day • Eyelid drooping (ptosis) • Double vision (diplopia) • Paralysis of eye movements	• Bulbar weakness resulting in dysarthria • Tiredness
Lambert-Eaton myasthenic syndrome	• Weakness improves throughout the day • Disruption of autonomic nervous system	• Diplopia • Ptosis • Lack of sweating (anhidrosis) • Orthostatic hypotension • Constipation

Contd…

Contd…

	Presenting characteristics of upper limb pain	Associated symptoms
Congenital myopathies (i.e. Duchenne muscular dystrophy and Becker's muscular dystrophy)	• Progressive muscular atrophy during adolescent development • Skeletal abnormalities	• Respiratory inadequacy
Degenerative arthritis of upper limb joints	• Discomfort • Pain of neck and/or back • Stiffness of neck and/or back	• Depression associated with disability • Nodules in joints are associated with rheumatoid arthritis (generally distal interphalangeal joints and cervical spine are unaffected)
Polymyalgia rheumatica fever	• Pain • Tenderness • Stiffness • Fever and headache	• Depression • Lethargy • Night sweats • Loss of appetite • Weight loss

(SLAP: Superior labral anterior to posterior).

Other diagnosis of peripheral neuropathy include nutritional deficiency, viral infection, Lyme disease, lead poisonings and other neurotoxins. This may be determined with a thorough history and laboratory workup.

of history especially potential mechanisms of injury, pathologic or traumatic. Remain cognizant of patient's experiences of limitations consistent with physical findings. Visual inspection of alignment and assessment of range of motion should be systematic, starting at the spine and working towards the periphery to ensure a comprehensive physical exam. If the patient has painful joints, let the patient move them gently to see how they manage or compensate for compromised range of motion. X-rays of recent traumatic injury to joints should be obtained prior to attempting range of motion tests. Long hair pulled up or aside and restrictive clothing should be removed prior to active and passive physical examination.

Begin by observing the general appearance, gait, and posture. Take notice of patient's ease in movement when walking, sitting and rising, and if applicable, ability to remove additional garments such as a jacket. Also observe for protective positioning of the upper limb. The use of an assistive device should be noted. Note any observable facial asymmetry, spasticity, dysarthria, or fasciculation as these are indications of motor neuron disease.

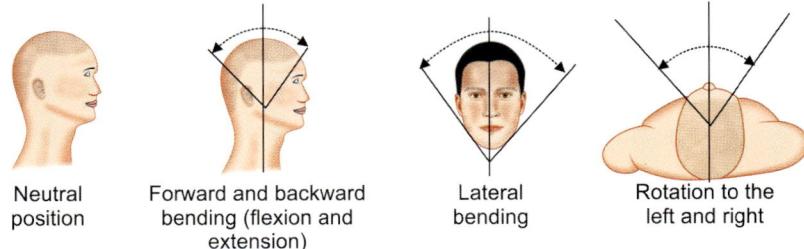

| Neutral position | Forward and backward bending (flexion and extension) | Lateral bending | Rotation to the left and right |

Fig. 3.1: Range of motion testing of the neck.

Note any bruising, ecchymosis, skin abrasions or other signs of trauma. Note any abnormalities of bony structures or soft tissue structures at joints upon palpation. During postural analysis, examine the patients resting head position and inclination of gaze. The patient should be able to look straight ahead with leveled shoulders. An elevated shoulder in relation to another may be indicative of scoliosis, muscle imbalance or glenohumeral instability.

Upon assessing the patient's cervical spine range of motion, the patient should be able to flex the neck (ask the patient to bring head to the chest and back to center) and extend the neck (ask the patient to lean head back and look at the ceiling) with ease (Fig. 3.1). The patient should be able to laterally flex the head (ask patient to bring head to one side of the shoulder and then the other) with ease and should be able to rotate head to the left and right (ask patient to look to the right and left) symmetrically with ease. Abnormal findings including limited range of motion, pain-limiting range of motion, asymmetry in range of movement for rotation or lateral bending, and fixed deformity in the sagittal or coronal plane may be indicative of nerve impingement.[2] The Spurling's test may be implemented to evaluate the patient for cervical root compression. Ask patient to extend the head and turn the head toward the affected side and apply downward pressure (Fig. 3.2). Pain arising from the neck in a dermatome may suggest cervical radiculopathy or cervical spondylitis.[1,3,14,15] Before assessing the integrity of the shoulder, check for tenderness to palpation of neck muscles or palpable neck masses. The presence of scars from prior surgery or injury should also be noted.

When performing physical examination of the shoulder, patient should be able to shrug the shoulders symmetrically. Tenderness or swelling upon palpitation of the sternoclavicular joint, clavicle, acromioclavicular (AC) joint, bicipital groove, periscapular area and around the subacromial bursa are suggestive of primary shoulder pathology. Check range of motion for forward flexion, abduction, internal and external rotation for passive and active range of motion. Move the arm while stabilizing the scapula with the other to help isolate glenohumeral joint during passive examination.

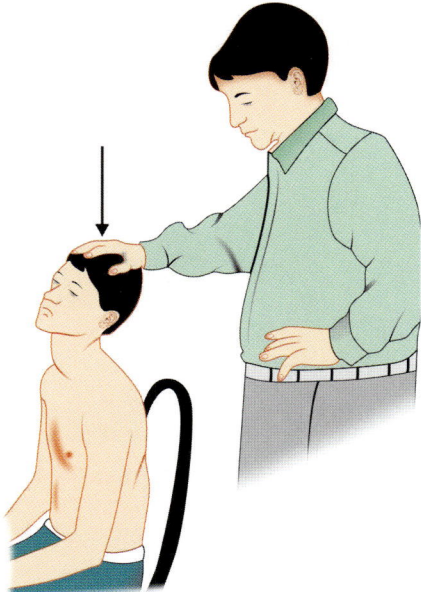

Fig. 3.2: Spurling's test is performed by extending the head and turning towards the affected side and applying downward pressure.

Improvement of symptoms with stabilization of the scapula is suggestive of scapular dyskinesis as is periscapular tenderness. If there is tenderness over the AC joint this is suggestive of arthritis or injury. Normal range of motion for abduction is up to 150° and adduction up to 30°. Forward shoulder flexion ranges from 0° to 180° and extension from 45° to 60°. Rotation of the shoulder should also be tested with the elbow flexed to 90° and should range from 0° to 90° in external rotation and 70°–90° in internal rotation (Fig. 3.3). Knowing expected range of motions can help assess for joint limitations during provocative maneuvers.

To assess whether the etiology of the patient's shoulder pain is of musculoskeletal origin, perform the cross body adduction test. Patients are asked to raise the affected arm to 90° and adduct the arm (cross the arm to reach the other clavicle). Motion with pain may be reflective of arthritis at the AC joint. Motion without pain rules out AC joint dysfunction and may indicate a rotator cuff impingement if the patient is experiencing shoulder pain.[9] Specific range of motion examinations may direct to a diagnosis of underlying pathology. The Neer's test can be implemented to detect rotator cuff tendon impingement under the coracoacromial notch.[11] While stabilizing the scapula with one hand, use the other to passively abduct the patient's pronated arm. Pain during forward flexion is a positive test. Typically patients with this abnormal finding will experience pain between 60° and 120° (Fig. 3.4). The Hawkins maneuver is useful in identifying a subacromial impingement or

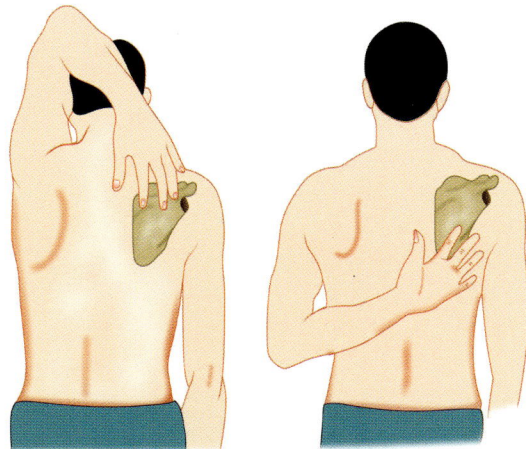

Fig. 3.3: Evaluation of range of motion of the shoulder in external rotation and internal rotation.

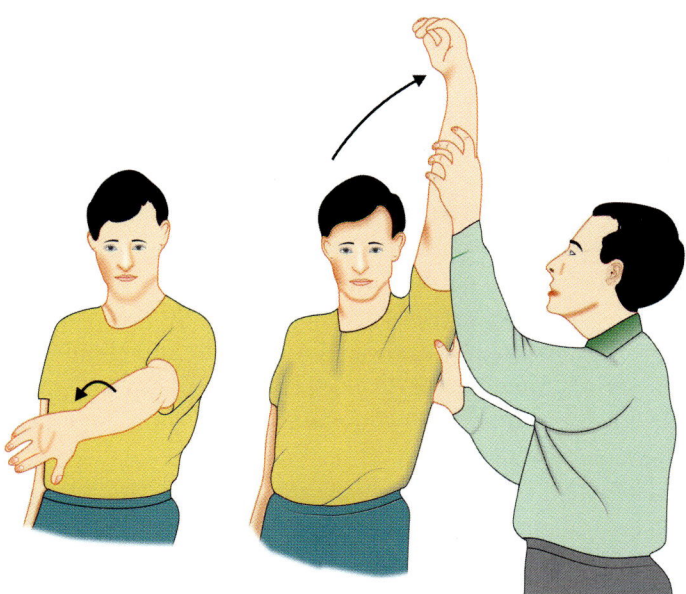

Fig. 3.4: Neer's test for impingement is performed by stabilizing the scapula and forward flexion of the patient's pronated arm.

tendonitis of the rotator cuff; this tests for the integrity of the infraspinatus (and teres minor muscle). A positive Hawkins sign is pain upon internally rotating the shoulder in question at 90° (in front of the chest); the arm should be stabilized while pushing down on the forearm. To improve the sensitivity of the Hawkins test, perform the infraspinatus test and painful arc test.[11] Position the patient's elbow so that it is at the side and at 90° with the humerus medially rotated

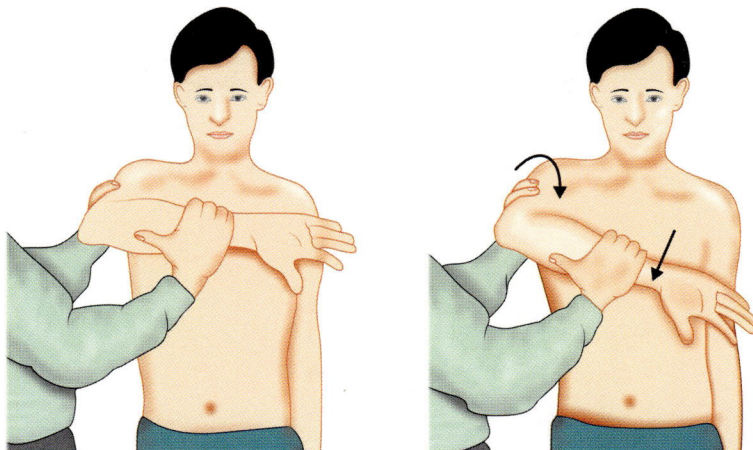

Fig. 3.5: Hawkins test is performed by internally rotating the arm with the shoulder at 90 degrees.

to 45°; apply rotational force medially (Fig. 3.5). Pain or inability to counter applied force is indicative of infraspinatus strain. Ask the patient to abduct the arm and bring it back to neutral, a positive painful arc test is pain between 60° and 120° of elevation during abduction. A drop arm test can be performed to diagnose a rotator cuff tear or supraspinatus strain.[23] Passively abduct the patient's arm in relation to the shoulder to 90°, and ask the patient to slowly lower the arm upon release. Failure to lower the arm in a controlled manner is a positive drop arm test. Note that control of arm motion above 90° abduction is by the deltoid muscle. Similarly the Jobe's test can be used to determine if the integrity of the supraspinatus is compromised. The patient is asked to abduct the arm and hold out his hand with the thumbs pointing down (as if emptying the contents of a can).[13] Provide downward pressure to test the strength of the patient's supraspinatus muscles (should provide substantial oppositional force) (Fig. 3.6). It is necessary to assess if there is injury to the labrum of the shoulder. Instruct patient to flex the arm to 90° with full extension of the elbow. Ask patient to internally rotate the arm so that the thumb points down and have patient resist downward force by the examiner. Ask patient to externally rotate the arm so that the thumb is up and provide downward force. Patient should be able to provide force upward. If the patient experiences pain, there may be associated clicking, and with downward pressure against the internally rotated arm and alleviation of pain when downward force is applied to an externally rotated arm, this may indicate damage of the labrum.

Swelling, warmth, erythema, pain with range of motion or an effusion can indicate infection. Focal posterior swelling over the olecranon with tenderness, warmth or erythema is consistent with bursitis in the absence of injury. Check for rashes or discoloration. Identify an excessive (cubitus valgus) or decreased

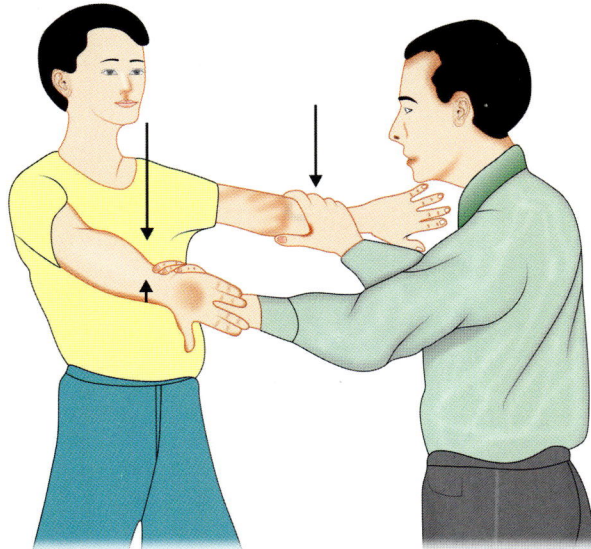

Fig. 3.6: Jobe's test is performed by applying downward force to the patient's abducted arm with the thumbs pointed down.

(cubitus varus) carrying angle of the elbow; females will have a larger expected carrying angle (Fig. 3.7). Assess the range of movement and integrity at the elbow joint with active and passive flexion and extension, and supination and pronation with flexed forearm. At the elbow, the patient should be able to extend the forearm to 0° and flex to 150°, and rotate the forearm with flexed elbow to 70° in pronation and 85° in supination. The patient should be able to perform movements with ease and without pain even with introduction of oppositional force. Patient may have weakness when tested with an opposing force if a neurologic injury is present or secondary to pain in the setting of trauma. Take note of crepitus or misalignment during range of motion.

Evaluate the muscles of the hand and wrist; the patient may present with abnormal contours of the hand with obvious signs of muscle wasting and/or deformities such as nodules. Identify pain or weakness by having the patient to sustain a tight and firm grasp on the examiner's two fingers. Ask patient to open and close the hand; patients should be able to do that 20 times in 10 seconds. Patients who are slow to open and close the hands at a rate lower than 20 times in 10 seconds, suggest stiffness or neurologic impairment from rheumatoid arthritis or cervical myelopathy respectively. In this test, patients may accelerate in the rate at which they open and close their hands, which is a hallmark sign of Lambert-Eaton myasthenic syndrome (patients with Lambert-Eaton will have progressive ease in motion when performing repetitive activities). Range of motion for ulnar and radial deviation is from 0° to 20° in the radial direction and 0°–30° in the ulnar direction. Extension

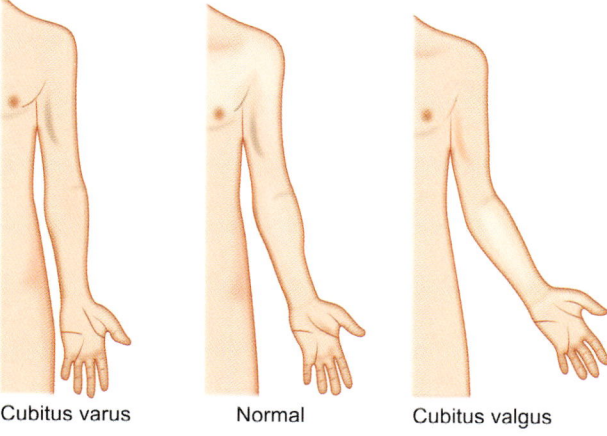

Cubitus varus   Normal   Cubitus valgus

Fig. 3.7: Carrying angles of the elbow.

and flexion of the hand at the wrist both range from 0° to 60° in their respective directions. Evaluate range of motion of the hand at wrist, thumb and digits; weakness and inability to flex or extend without pain is indicative of pathology. Patient should be able to extend and flex the wrist and digits and oppose the thumb. Successful execution of full range of motion at the thumb at the metacarpophalangeal joint should continue up to 60° (flexion) and at the interphalangeal joints to 80°. Flexion of the digits at the metacarpophalangeal joints should continue up to 90° and extension up to 30°. Abduction of the digits at the metacarpophalangeal joints should continue up to 25°.[30]

If patient experiences upper limb pain at rest and throughout physical exam, a diagnosis of thoracic outlet syndrome may be considered. There are controversies in regards to diagnosis (and management) of thoracic syndrome as compression may be of vascular, neurogenic, or a combination of both in origin.[27] Patient can present with a range of symptoms in regards to severity and progression of the compression. A diagnosis of thoracic outlet syndrome is determined when there is compressive pressure on the nerves and blood vessels that travel in the space between the clavicle and first rib.[28] Start the patient with an elevated arm stress test. Ask patient to raise both arms over the head (at 90° abduction) and to open and close fists for a few minutes. In thoracic outlet syndrome, there is compression of the brachial plexus and/or blood vessels as they leave through the thoracic outlet between the clavicle and the first rib to innervate and supply the arm respectively (Fig. 3.8). Patients may complain of a vague pain that is over the neck, shoulder, arm and lateral hand region. There may be swelling or redness of the arm; patients may also feel cold to the touch distally. Overhead actions recreate or exacerbate symptoms consistent with thoracic outlet syndrome findings (i.e. generalized aching sensation in the neck and/or arm with pain, numbness or tingling in the forearm that may extend to lateral digits). Visual

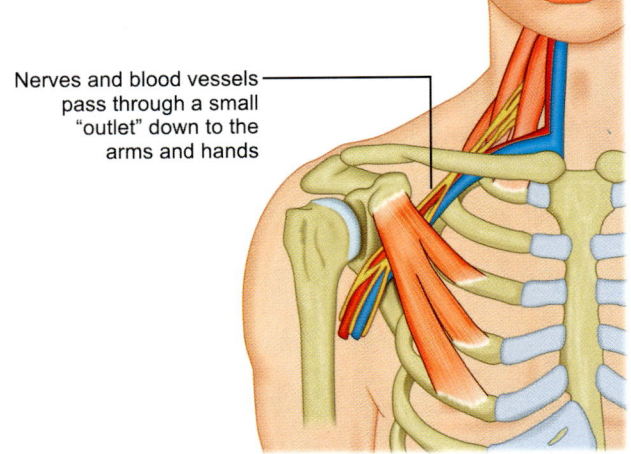

Nerves and blood vessels pass through a small "outlet" down to the arms and hands

Fig. 3.8: Brachial plexus and blood vessels traveling under the clavicle to the arm.

inspection for cyanosis, edema, irregularities in the supraclavicular fossa, and muscular atrophy of the hand is common. Further diagnostic measures with X-rays, computed tomography (CT) scan, magnetic resonance imaging (MRI) and ultrasound may be necessary. Non-invasive ultrasound imaging should be used first to determine if there is occlusion to the subclavian artery or potential bony and/or soft tissue abnormalities. Additional X-ray, CT or MRI with arteriography/venography may be taken to further examine the integrity of the subclavian artery, and identify the location of vascular compression and related pathology. Injection of local anesthetic to the anterior scalene muscle may be considered as a diagnostic measure; relief of pain may indicate thoracic outlet syndrome.

When evaluating a patient who presents with generalized and widespread musculoskeletal pain, who can perform active and passive motions with relative ease, ask the patient to elaborate more about the presentation and origin of the pain and associated symptoms. Patients may describe widespread musculoskeletal pain along with feeling a sense of fatigue, delay in cognitive activities, sleep dysfunction, stiffness, anxiety and depression. Through eliminating other potential systemic neuromuscular and musculoskeletal diseases by physical examination and laboratory testing, and obtaining a throughout history, the examiner may the examiner may diagnose the patient with fibromyalgia.[21]

NEUROLOGIC EXAMINATIONS

When patients present with upper limb pain, it is important to maintain awareness of pyramidal tract and myotome and dermatome distribution of spinal nerves to help identify origin of symptoms (pain and/or weakness). During physical examination, observe signs of damage to upper and lower motor neurons. Spasticity, clonus or hyperreflexia are indicative of upper motor neuron damage, whereas flaccid paralysis is often associated with lower motor neuron damage. Special attention to facial symmetry, tongue deviations and dysarthria should be noted as they may be indicative of CNS damage. To screen for sensory deficits, feel the lateral aspect of the arm at the elbow (C5), the thumb (C6), the middle digit (C7), the fifth digit (C8) and medial elbow (T1) with light touch and pinprick for two point discrimination. Altered sensation suggests peripheral neuropathy from medical causes or nerve compression from the brachial plexus or CNS injury. The brachial plexus comprises the dermatome and cutaneous distribution of upper limb (Figs. 3.9 and 3.10). Note that C3 and C4 spinal nerves have some sensory innervation that start at the base of the neck and extends out over the shoulders, respectively. The branches of the brachial plexus are musculocutaneous (C5, 6, 7), axillary (C5, 6), median (C5, 6, 7, 8 and T1), radial (C5, 6, 7, 8 and T1) and ulnar (C8 and T1). The musculocutaneous branch provides sensory innervation to the lateral forearm. The axillary nerve provides sensory innervation of the skin over the lower deltoid down to the upper forearm. The median nerve provides sensory innervation of the lateral aspect of the palm and the lateral three and half digits. The radial nerve provides sensory innervation to the posterior aspect of the forearm, the dorsal surface of the lateral side of the hand and the lateral three and half digits. The ulnar nerve provides sensory innervation to the anterior and posterior surfaces of the medial one and half fingers and medial palmar surface.[29] Perform deep tendon reflex assessments such as biceps reflex (C5), brachioradialis reflex (C6), tricep reflex (C7), as well as Spurling's and Hoffman's test. The Hoffman's test is primarily used to evaluate the integrity of corticospinal tract and is often present in the setting of cervical myelopathy or other cord disease. When considering a diagnosis of cervical myelopathy, further imaging studies may be useful.[10] The examiner will attempt to elicit a response by tapping down on the nail/terminal phalanx of the third digit. No flexion of other digits should be seen. Hyporeflexia during deep tendon reflex testing indicates peripheral nerve injury or disease. Hyperreflexia and pathologic reflexes are indicative of upper motor neuron disease/CNS pathology.

Imaging Studies

X-Ray/Radiographs

Pending the pattern of exam and the history, imaging may include antero-posterior (AP), lateral, flexion, extension and open mouth views. A complete radiographic series of the shoulder including anteroposterior (AP), lateral,

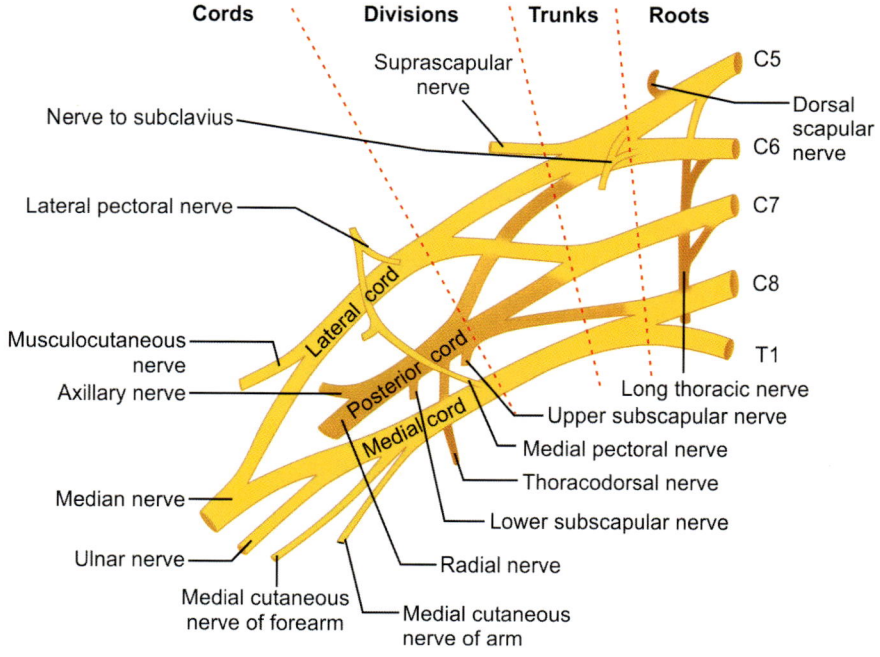

Fig. 3.9: Brachial plexus.

internal and external rotation, scapular Y and an axillary view are recommended. The basic radiographic evaluation of the elbow includes AP, lateral and oblique views. The hand and wrist also require AP, lateral and oblique views with special views to evaluate the carpal tunnel/hamate hook and scaphoid. Radiographs in the cervical spine can demonstrate bony injury or instability on the flexion-extension view. In addition the presence of arthritic changes, infection, or malignancy affecting the bone can be appreciated. Soft tissues are not to be neglected as prevertebral soft tissue swelling, air, calcified masses and other irregularities are often captured on plain films. In addition, distortions of normal anatomical structures such as the trachea can be appreciated.

In evaluation of extremity films, careful evaluation of the soft tissue can reveal joint effusion, soft tissue masses, or collections. In general bone osteopenia with overall mineralization can be appreciated. Focal osteopenia is noted with concern for infection or infiltrative lesions. Similarly abnormal patterns of increased bone density must be explained. Arthritis with joint space narrowing, subchondral sclerosis, and cystic changes, as well as fracture, and bone lesions are often readily appreciated. In the glenohumeral joint, the congruency is assessed on perpendicular views. All views must show a congruent joint and an axillary lateral or scapular Y view are necessary. Maintenance of normal

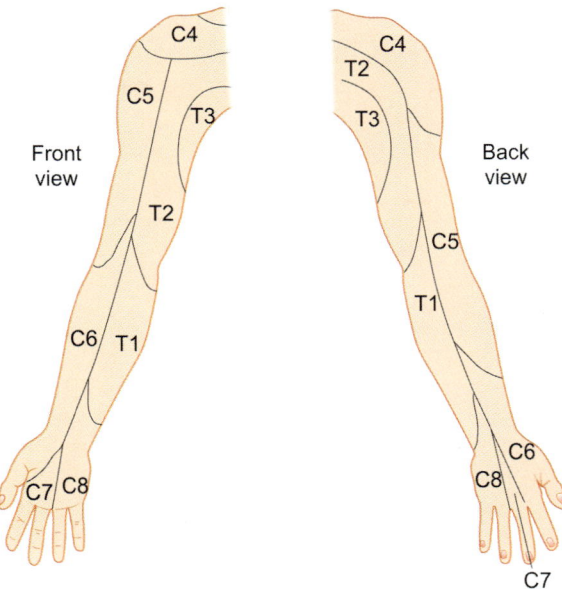

Fig. 3.10: Dermatomes of the arm.

relationships of the AC, coracoacromial, glenohumeral and scapulothoracic joints can be appreciated on an appropriate radiographic series (Fig. 3.11).

Computed Tomography

Computed tomography scan is indicated to evaluate three-dimensional structure of bone as well as cross-sectional imaging in high spatial resolution.[4] Sensitivity and specificity for fracture, as well as bone lesions is very high. Increased cross-sectional density in the soft tissue is readily appreciated such as ossification of the posterior longitudinal ligament. Isolated ligamentous injury may be missed as can hematoma, soft tissue lesions, or presence of infection. Contrast CT imaging may be requested when the study is to evaluate for malignancy or infection.

Magnetic Resonance Imaging

Magnetic resonance imaging allows evaluation of the soft tissue elements with high sensitivity for pathology at moderate spatial resolution.[4,5] Spin sequences can be varied allowing for delineation of most pathologies present in soft tissue. In the case of infection or malignancy, contrast may be helpful should the patient be able to tolerate exposure. Ligamentous injury is readily appreciated as well as edema, inflammation, soft tissue masses, fluid collections, and the presence of scar tissue. Spinal cord injury as well as root, plexus, or peripheral nerve impingement can also be ascertained.

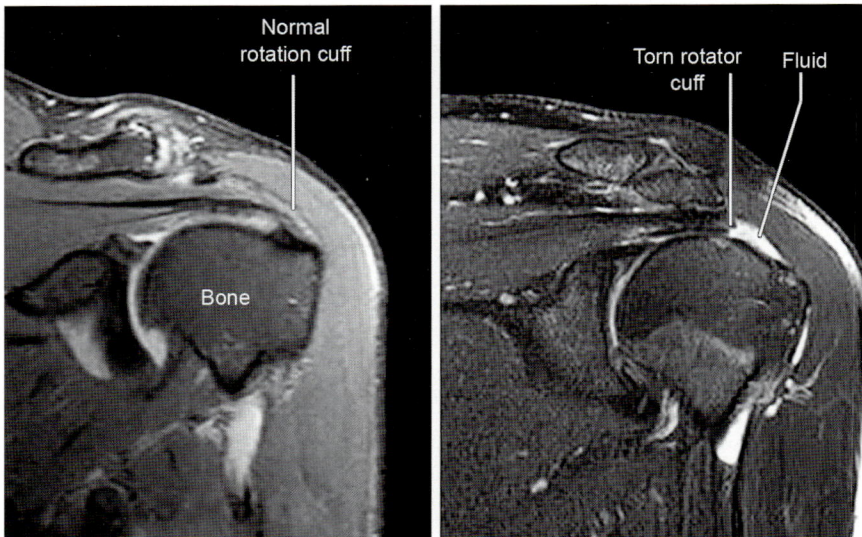

Fig. 3.11: Coronal sections of a normal shoulder MRI and a rotator cuff tear.

Ultrasound

Ultrasound is a minimally invasive technique that can access joint and tendon movements.[26] It can detect tears, calcification and fluid within a joint. This test is useful in patients who are unable to undergo MRI such as patients with metal implants or pacemakers.

Further Workup

Nerve Conduction Velocity and EMG Lab Testing

Electromyography and nerve conduction studies are used to evaluate muscle weakness and wasting through quantifying muscle activity and sensory symptoms. Electrodes are placed over the area of interest, generally over areas of motor, sensory or mixed nerves. Generally the electrodes are placed on the skin overlying the surface of muscle bellies in question.[12] Through the use of mild electrical stimulations, muscle and nerve response can be observed and recorded. Similarly, a needle electrode may be utilized to record muscle activity and detect any involuntary muscle spasms.[6,8]

Electromyography tests are particularly helpful in diagnosing peripheral neuropathies.[7] These results can not only help to locate the potential origin of patients' muscular symptoms, but also help to determine whether the pathology is that of mononeuropathy, polyneuropathy, polyradiculopathy, plexopathy, motor neuropathy or sensory neuropathy of the dorsal root ganglion (DRG).

Evaluation of upper and lower extremities often involves placing the electrode over the median and ulnar nerve, and the tibial and peroneal nerve respectively. EMG studies can aid in evaluating the prognosis of a traumatic nerve injury by observing conduction failure, axonal degeneration, and the compound muscle action potential (CMAP) amplitude. EMG tests can also be used to observe the progress of muscle and nerve function of a patient following invasive and non-invasive therapeutic approaches to determine if management of neuromuscular junction disease has been beneficial. EMG is not necessarily a definitive diagnostic tool; other laboratory tests and physical examinations may be used to eliminate other potential diagnosis.

Nerve conduction studies are utilized to exclude peripheral disease from amyotrophic lateral sclerosis (ALS). EMG can be used to diagnose a patient with ALS even before its gross clinical manifestations. ALS patients usually have normal sensory findings with observable fibrillation potentials and decreased recruitment. Decreases in CMAP amplitude are often observed.[22,31]

Genetic Testing

Some conditions for affecting sensory and motor changes in the extremity are genetic, such as Charcot-Marie-Tooth (CMT) disease. CMT characteristically affects the lower extremity but this and other genetic neuropathies can be present in upper extremity as well. Mutations in the *DMPK* gene (myotonic dystrophy type 1) and *CNBP* gene (myotonic dystrophy type 2) can be detected on genetic testing. Congenital myotonic dystrophy affects 1 in 8,000. Patients with myotonic dystrophy experience prolonged muscle contraction, with inability to relax certain muscles after use. Myotonic dystrophy is also characterized by progressive muscle wasting.

Lab Workup

Infection is often on the differential diagnosis, and if so, complete blood count (CBC) with differential, C-reactive protein (CRP), erythrocyte sedimentation rate (ESR) and more recently p-calcitonin are sensitive markers for infection depending on the acuity and severity. If peripheral nerve pathology is suspected, further testing may include a CBC, ESR, glucose levels, vitamin B12 and Lyme titers. Blood tests for antibodies against acetylcholine receptors and calcium channels or other potential antigens characteristic of neuromuscular disorders should be obtained. CSF samples with elevated protein and immunoglobulin may indicate neurological pathology.

CONCLUSION

When patient presents with upper limb pain or weakness, careful assessment based on thorough history and range of motion will help to determine underlying pathologies. While the most common cause of upper limb pain is due to muscular strain, special attention to patient responsiveness during deep tendon reflex tests and provocative maneuvers help to identify neurologic damage. Visual inspection for cyanosis, edema, irregularities and muscular atrophy of the neck and upper limb musculature is necessary. Further diagnostic measures with X-rays, CT scan, MRI and ultrasound may be beneficial in confirming a diagnosis. Non-invasive ultrasound imaging should be used first to determine the presence of occlusion to the arteries or compression by potential bony and/or soft tissue abnormalities. Additional X-ray, CT or MRI with arteriography/venography may be obtained to further examine the integrity of the major upper limb vasculature, and identify the location of arterial compression and related pathology. Introduction of local anesthetics to neck and upper limb muscles may be used as a diagnostic measure and a temporary control of pain. Lab work (including genetic testing) may help to identify less common causes of upper limb pain and weakness such as muscular dystrophy, autoimmune diseases, nutritional deficiencies, neurotoxins and Lyme disease.

REFERENCES

1. Carette S, Fehlings MG. Cervical radiculopathy. N Engl J Med. 2005;353(4):392-9.
2. Slaven EJ, Mathers J. Differential diagnosis of shoulder and cervical pain: a case report. J Man Manip Ther. 2010;18(4):191-6.
3. Chaudhary SB, Hullinger H, Vives MJ. Management of acute spinal fractures in ankylosing spondylitis. ISRN Rheumatol. 2011;2011:150484.
4. Gundry CR, Heithoff KB. Imaging evaluation of patients with spinal deformity. Orthop Clin North Am. 1994;25(2):247-64.
5. Como JJ, Thompson MA, Anderson JS, et al. Is magnetic resonance imaging essential in clearing the cervical spine in obtunded patients with blunt trauma? J Trauma. 2007;63(3):544-9.
6. Pozzo M, Merlo E, Farina D, et al. Muscle-fiber conduction velocity estimated from surface EMG signals during explosive dynamic contractions. Muscle Nerve. 2004;29(6):823-33.
7. Wijesekera LC, Leigh PN. Amyotrophic lateral sclerosis. Orphanet J Rare Dis. 2009;4:3.
8. Chichkova RI, Katzin L. (2010) EMG and nerve conduction studies in clinical practice. [online] Available from practicalneurology.com/2010/02/emg-and-nerve-conduction-studies-in-clinical-practice/. [Accessed July, 2015].
9. Kappe T, Knappe K, Elsharkawi M, et al. Predictive value of preoperative clinical examination for subacromial decompression in impingement syndrome. Knee Surg Sports Traumatol Arthrosc. 2015;23(2):443-8.
10. Rhee JM, Heflin JA, Hamasaki T, et al. Prevalence of physical signs in cervical myelopathy: a prospective, controlled study. Spine (Phila Pa 1976). 2009;34(9): 890-5.
11. Michener LA, Walsworth MK, Doukas WC, et al. Reliability and diagnostic accuracy of 5 physical examination tests and combination of tests for subacromial impingement. Arch Phys Med Rehabil. 2009;90(11):1898-903.
12. Mesin L, Merletti R, Rainoldi A. Surface EMG: the issue of electrode location. J Electromyogr Kinesiol. 2009;19(5):719-26.
13. Forbush SW, White DM, Smith W. THE comparison of the empty can and full can techniques and a new diagonal horizontal adduction test for supraspinatus

muscle testing using cross-sectional analysis through ultrasonography. Int J Sports Phys Ther. 2013;8(3):237-47.

14. Shabat S, Leitner Y, David R, et al. The correlation between Spurling test and imaging studies in detecting cervical radiculopathy. J Neuroimaging. 2012;22(4):375-8.

15. Tong HC, Haig AJ, Yamakawa K. The Spurling test and cervical radiculopathy. Spine. 2002;27(2):156-9.

16. Meriggioli MN, Sanders DB. Autoimmune myasthenia gravis: emerging clinical and biological heterogeneity. Lancet Neurol. 2009;8(5):475-90.

17. Ahonen A, Pyhtinen J, Hokkanen E, et al. Cerebrospinal fluid protein findings in cervical syndromes classified by myelography, and in multiple sclerosis. Acta Neurol Scand. 1982;66(3):369-77.

18. Edwards II CC, Riew KD, Anderson PA, et al. Cervical myelopathy: current diagnostic and treatment strategies. Spine J. 2003;3(1):68-81.

19. Truumees E, Herkowitz HN. Cervical spondylotic myelopathy and radiculopathy. Instr Course Lect. 2009;49:339-60.

20. Wu X, Wang J, Liu Y, et al. Clinical presentation and differential diagnosis of Lambert-Eaton myasthenic syndrome. Neurosci Riyadh Saudi Arab. 2013;18(2):169-72.

21. Goldenberg DL. Diagnosis and differential diagnosis of fibromyalgia. Am J Med. 2009 Dec;122(12 Suppl):S14-21.

22. Fuglsang-Frederiksen A. Diagnostic criteria for amyotrophic lateral sclerosis (ALS). Clin Neurophysiol. 2008;119(3):495-6.

23. Lansdown DA, Feeley BT. Evaluation and treatment of rotator cuff tears. Phys Sportsmed. 2012;40(2):73-86.

24. Rossier AB, Foo D, Shillito J, et al. Posttraumatic cervical syringomyelia. Incidence, clinical presentation, electrophysiological studies, syrinx protein and results of conservative and operative treatment. Brain J Neurol. 1985;108(Pt 2):439-61.

25. Hoang PD, Gandevia SC, Herbert RD. Prevalence of joint contractures and muscle weakness in people with multiple sclerosis. Disabil Rehabil. 2014; 36(19):1588-93.

26. Blankstein A. Ultrasound in the diagnosis of clinical orthopedics: the orthopedic stethoscope. World J Orthop. 2011;2(2):13-24.

27. Hooper TL, Denton K, McGalliard MK, et al. Thoracic outlet syndrome: a controversial clinical condition. Part 1: anatomy and clinical examination/diagnosis. J Mann Manip Ther. 2010;18(2):74-83.

28. Laulan J, Fouquet B, Rodiax C, et al. Thoracic outlet syndrome: definition, aetiological factors, diagnosis, management and occupational impact. J Occup Rehabil. 2011;21(3):366-73.

29. Moore KL, Agur AMR, Dalley AF. Essential Clinical Anatomy, 4th edition. Baltimore, MD: Lippincott Williams & Wilkins; 2011.

30. Bain GI, Polites N, Higgs BG, et al. (2014) The functional range of motion of the finger joints. J Hand Surg Eur Vol. 2015;40(4):406-11.

31. Van der Hoeven JH, Zwarts MJ, Van Weerden TW. Muscle fiber conduction velocity in amyotrophic lateral sclerosis and traumatic lesions of the plexus brachialis. Electroencephalogr Clin Neurophysiol. 1993;89(5):304-10.

CHAPTER 4

Cervical versus Shoulder/ Periscapular Pain

Christie Stawicki, Tristan Fried, Loren Mead, Sarah Nyirjesy, John D Koerner, Alexander R Vaccaro

CHIEF COMPLAINT/HISTORY

In a patient with cervical spine or shoulder pathology, the chief complaint will be of pain in the region from the neck to the upper arm. Neck and shoulder pain are two of the most common complaints of all patients. An epidemiological study surveying the prevalence of musculoskeletal pains found that shoulder pain was the third most common reported type of pain at a prevalence of 16% and was only surpassed by low back and knee pain.[1] Neck pain was the fourth most prevalent at 14%. The incidence increases with patient age until about 65 years when their frequency tends to plateau. As a majority of the musculoskeletal pains are reported in the working population, they contribute significantly to the spending of healthcare dollars as well as lost worker productivity.[2] In addition to the chief complaint of pain, there can be a variety of other complaints caused by cervical spine and shoulder pathology leading to weakness as well numbness in the neck, upper back, and upper extremities. With many potential sources of cervical spine and shoulder pathology, a distinct injury may have been the original cause of the pain, and therefore understanding the initial injury could help to diagnose the pathology. Certainly many patients will simultaneously have concomitant shoulder and cervical pathology, and the overlap can be difficult to distinguish. It is important to consider the timing of treatment in patients with concomitant shoulder and cervical pathology. For example, deltoid function is crucial for rehabilitation of rotator cuff injuries, and if compromised by cervical radiculopathy (CR), should be treated prior to rotator cuff interventions.

Understanding the presentation of symptoms is an essential clue to the etiology, specifically activities that exacerbate or relieve the pain. Careful consideration to one's vocational activities can be helpful. In addition, the quality of the symptoms described by the patient can be very informative. Descriptors such as feelings of instability, catching, or immobility frequently refer to a joint problem. Nerve pain is frequently described as burning, sharp, shooting and electrical. Tendonitis pain is frequently described as aching, dull, and diffuse.[3]

When it comes to the cervical spine and shoulder, it is important to recognize and consider other pathology that is not present in the area but is, in fact, referred pain from an internal organ or body system. Pain associated with chest discomfort, dyspnea, nausea, diaphoresis, dizziness, a racing heart, or jaw pain should prompt concern regarding referred pain from coronary artery, pulmonary embolism, or gastrointestinal origins.

DIFFERENTIAL DIAGNOSIS

In order to treat pain correctly, one must first differentiate between the etiology of cervical spine pain and shoulder pain. This can be challenging as the areas are not only in close proximity but can share muscles, nerves and vessels. In general, within each region there are three major types of pathology that can be experienced: musculoskeletal, nervous, or vascular.

For the shoulder, the most common musculoskeletal pathologies include: degenerative joint disease, rotator cuff pain, impingement, and adhesive capsulitis. Pain is a frequent complaint most often without true weakness or numbness. However, shoulder pain can lead to weakness caused by pain inhibition and disuse atrophy. The patient may describe the shoulder joint as "catching" with motion or as being "frozen" with the inability to perform a motion. Shoulder pathology is also more common when pain is with overhead activity or with night pain. Pain in the deltoid region is more often rotator cuff, but pain in the periscapular region can be either from the shoulder or cervical spine. Pain radiating past the elbow is also usually of cervical etiology.

Neck pain may be acute and, at times, transient as in a muscular strain and sprain. This may be associated with staying in a prolonged uncomfortable position or perhaps having a sudden cervical flexion/extension injury. Chronic neck stiffness and discomfort is frequently associated with underlying arthritic disks and facet degeneration. In CR, key symptoms may include pain and sensory loss which may radiate down a specific dermatome. In addition, there may be weakness that may follow in the corresponding myotome. Spondylosis leading to foraminal encroachment is the most common cause of radicular pain.[4] Any acute pain associated with trauma needs to be evaluated for underlying cervical fracture or instability. Nerve injuries can include brachial plexus injuries, radiculopathy or specific nerve entrapments.

Vascular injuries and syndromes are generally less common. They are caused by the partial occlusion of arteries and veins. These may accompany a history of trauma. They can lead to pain, swelling, cyanotic limb coloring, weakness and non-dermatomal sensory loss. The acute onset of vascular origins of pain should initiate a prompt workup as these symptoms could progress to permanent functional losses.

In assessing the patient it is important to address the patient's past medical history specifically asking about their occupation and injury history. Symptoms that can be concerning for an underlying cancer or infection may include fever, night sweats, weight loss, intractable night pain, and lymphadenopathy. When examining the patient with neck pain one must ask questions that might indicate myelopathy such as abnormal gait, decreased balance, or difficulty manipulating small objects.[5] Findings of acute cervical myelopathy also should initiate an urgent evaluation as the symptoms may progress to permanent dysfunction.

WORKUP

The main anatomical cause of CR is nerve root compression as the cervical spinal nerves exit the spinal cord and progresses towards the neural foramen[6] (Fig. 4.1). Most important in diagnosing CR is a patient's history,[7] as noted by complaints of arm pain and paresthesias of specific dermatomes. Nerve compression may be present on different cervical vertebral levels, each demonstrating specific symptoms.[6]

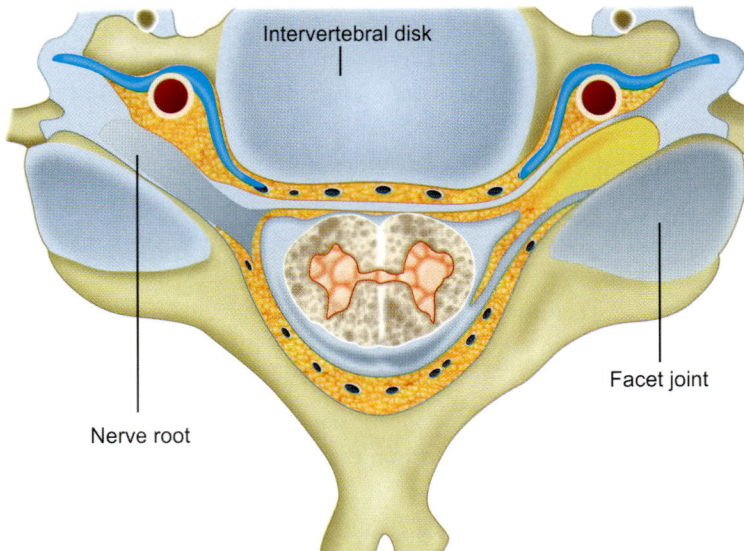

Fig. 4.1: Axial representation of C5 vertebra looking cephalad to caudal.
Source: Caridi JM et al. (2011).

Physical Exam

- Observe the patient through full neck range of motion including flexion, extension, rotation and lateral bending. Observe any abnormal resting posture, which may include tilting of the head and neck away from the affected area.[8]
- Decreased range of motion is usually observed in lateral bending, rotation, and extension as a result of narrowing of the foramen.[6] Note that passive shoulder motion is generally maintained in cases of CR.[9]
- Ipsilateral pain is usually caused by compression of a nerve root at the neural foramen.[6] Normally, lateral bending of the neck away from the affected side will ameliorate painful symptoms; however, continued pain may still occur after lateral bending of neck away from affected side which may indicate a herniated disk impinging on nerve root rather than spondylosis.[11]
- Sensory examination may show a decrease in sensation in specific dermatomes, as noted by potentiated response to light touch and pinprick.[10]

Palpation

- Palpation of cervical paraspinal muscles may elicit soreness, particularly on the ipsilateral side of compressed nerve roots, medial scapula, and proximal arm region.
- Isolated tenderness to palpation over bony prominences (medial or lateral epicondyle) will more likely be due to local inflammation rather than of cervical origin.
- Diffuse tenderness to palpation in multiple areas should alert the clinician to the possibility of fibromyalgia.

Motor

- Manual motor testing should be performed on all patients with suspected cervical or shoulder pathology and may demonstrate weakness in specific muscle groups. Patients with shoulder pathology may have weakness in the deltoid or biceps, which is why a complete exam including reflexes, sensory, and provocative maneuvers must be performed. Specific motor testing is described in Table 4.1.

Deep Tendon Reflexes

Reflex testing should always be performed in comparison to the contra-lateral asymptomatic side, noting any diminished reflexes. Hyperreflexia is indicative of an upper motor neuron lesion such as myelopathy from cord compression. There is significant variability in reflex response based

Table 4.1: Nerve roots and associated dermatomes, motor functions and reflexes.

Nerve root	Described pain, diminished sensation	Motor weakness	Reflex deficits
C5	Lateral arm	Shoulder abduction Elbow flexion	Biceps brachii
C6	Lateral forearm, thumb, index, radial half of middle finger	Wrist extension Elbow flexion	Brachioradialis
C7	Middle finger	Elbow extension, wrist flexion, finger extension	Triceps
C8	Ring and small finger, medial forearm	Finger flexion	None
T1	Medial upper forearm, arm	Finger abduction	None

on patient age, size, and comorbidities, which emphasizes the importance of comparing to the contralateral side. Reflexes in the upper extremity are described in Table 4.1.

Sensation

Patients may describe pain or numbness and tingling that corresponds to a particular dermatome, or have diminished sensation on light touch or pinprick exam. Upper cervical spine pathology may present with jaw pain or occipital headaches (C1, C2), or upper neck and trapezial pain (C3, C4).[6,9,18] Characteristic dermatomes of the upper extremity are further described in Table 4.1.

Provocative Tests

Cervical spine:
- The Spurling's test (ST) involves neck extension, rotation and lateral bending towards the side of pain with axial compression. This causes narrowing of the affected foramen and reproduction of the patient's symptoms. This test is very specific, but not necessarily sensitive.[19]
- The upper limb tension test (ULTT) is the upper extremity equivalent to the straight leg raise for the lumbar spine. While there are many variations of this maneuver, they all attempt to exacerbate CR symptoms by stretching the implicated nerve root. The patient lies in the supine position and the ipsilateral extremity is abducted with the elbow extended and forearm supinated, with the wrist and fingers extended while the neck is turned to the contralateral side.
- The shoulder abduction test involves placement of the palm of the ipsilateral hand on top of the head, which will relieve radicular pain by opening the foramen of the involved nerve roots.

Shoulder:

- There are numerous provocative maneuvers to test for shoulder pathology. While this list may not be exhaustive, the clinician should be familiar with the more sensitive tests to rule out shoulder pathology. Observation of asymmetric atrophy around the scapula and shoulder could be due to peripheral nerve compression. The suprascapular nerve can be compressed at the suprascapular notch or spinoglenoid notch and cause pain and atrophy. Weakness of the infraspinatus may be observed with external rotation with the elbow at the side.
- The Neer impingement sign, evaluated by passive elevation of the arm (between abduction and forward flexion) while the examiner stabilizes the ipsilateral scapula, is considered positive for subacromial impingement when patient experiences pain.
- The Hawkins sign for subacromial impingement is performed by flexing the shoulder and elbow to 90°, followed by internal rotation. Pain during passive internal rotation is considered a positive sign. Both Hawkins and Neer signs are highly sensitive but not specific for the presence of shoulder impingement.[9]
- The Jobe test involves abducting the shoulder 90° and forward flexion 30° with internal rotation of the arms. Apply downward force on the arms while patient resists; weakness is indicative of a rotator cuff tear or impingement.
- The cross body adduction test is performed by forward elevation of the arm and passive adduction towards the contralateral shoulder. Pain over the acromioclavicular (AC) joint is indicative of pathology.
- Yergason's sign is positive with pain in the bicipital groove when resisted supination is attempted with the elbow flexed 90° and the forearm pronated.
- Wright's test for thoracic outlet syndrome is performed by externally rotating and abducting the patient's arm while turning the head away. Loss of the radial pulse is indicative of thoracic outlet syndrome.
- Scapular winging can be detected by having the patient push against a wall with their arms forward flexed 90°. If the inferior border of the scapula migrates medially, pathology in the serratus anterior or long thoracic nerve is likely. If the scapula migrates laterally, the trapezius or spinal accessory nerve is likely involved.

Imaging Studies

Along with physical examination, radiographic imaging and electrodiagnostic studies can assist the clinician to distinguish cervical from shoulder pathology. Because dermatomal arm pain alone is not specific in identifying the pathologic level in patients with CR, further evaluation including radiographs, magnetic resonance imaging (MRI), computed tomography (CT), or CT myelography, is suggested before surgical decompression.[12] Imaging of the shoulder should also be obtained if there is suspicion for concomitant pathology.

Radiographic imaging can assist in evaluating the alignment of the cervical spine, in addition to identifying degenerative changes as well as fracture. Radiographs of the shoulder commonly demonstrate osteophyte formation, joint space narrowing, and sclerosis.[10] Shoulder films can also display superior head migration, arthritis of the glenohumeral and AC joints, and rounding and/or sclerosis of the greater tuberosity. An axillary view is helpful to visualize arthritis and anterior/posterior translation. The outlet view is best to evaluate acromial morphology. Ultrasound can be used to evaluate rotator cuff, but results are subjective to the experience of the operator.

Magnetic resonance imaging is recommended for the confirmation of correlative compressive lesions (disk herniation and spondylosis) in cervical spine patients who have failed a course of conservative therapy, and who may be candidates for interventional or surgical treatment.[13] Advantages of MRI include superior evaluation of soft tissue compressive lesions, better evaluation of spinal cord pathology, and the ability to avoid ionizing radiation. On the contrary, disadvantages include contraindications with ferromagnetic implants around vital structures, image quality sensitive to metal implants, and difficulty of distinguishing soft versus hard disk. MRI must be used to confirm physical exam findings and history given the high incidence of false positives. Evaluation for signal change in the spinal cord can illustrate irreversible damage (myelomalacia).

Computed tomography myelography is suggested for the evaluation of patients with clinical symptoms or signs that are discordant with MRI findings (e.g. foraminal compression that may not be identified on MRI). CT myelography better delineates soft versus hard disk, as opposed to other methods. For patients who have a contraindication to MRI, CT myelography is primarily utilized.

Due to high sensitivity and specificity, MRI is accurate in determining the size of the tear and status of rotator cuff muscles, in addition to possible soft tissue causes of impingement, and the presence of other shoulder pathology. Evaluation of rotator cuff for fatty infiltration and atrophy should be indicated only if surgery is to be considered. MRI of the shoulder should be performed to identify potential compressive lesions and to rule out rotator cuff tear.[10] MRI may detect muscle signal abnormalities; however, it should not stand alone as basis for clinical diagnosis. In asymptomatic individuals, a significant rate of positive findings is common.

FURTHER WORKUP

Electromyography (EMG) can assist in distinguishing radiculopathies from peripheral entrapment disorders. According to the American Association of Neuromuscular and Electrodiagnostic Medicine, in a meta-analysis of nine studies, EMG had a sensitivity of 50–71% for the diagnosis of CR.[14] EMG provides sensitivity and specificity which assists in ruling out other disorders. Reported sensitivities from unblinded studies resulted in variations of 30–95%. EMG results were compared with data on root compression verified during surgery, or obtained by MRI or clinical examination.[15] As most C6 muscles are also innervated by C5 or C7, identifying a C6 radiculopathy by EMG data alone is difficult. Paraspinal muscle examination is more sensitive, however, from a technical standpoint, more challenging with false-positive results in elderly patient populations.[15] In an attempt to determine the stage and severity of the root compression, needle examination can also be utilized. Abnormal spontaneous activity may appear in severe cases 3 weeks after onset of symptoms illustrating axon loss. In cases of chronic radiculopathy, neurogenic recruitment patterns can be seen as a result of collateral sprouting. The critical role of neurophysiological examination is to rule out other conditions including median or ulnar nerve entrapment with nerve conduction studies.

Additionally, selective nerve root block (SNRB) injection can predict surgical outcome for CR, however, they can lead to catastrophic outcomes. Spinal cord injury and cerebrovascular accident can result if not performed correctly.[16] SNRB with specific dosing and technique protocols may be considered in the evaluation of patients with CR and compressive lesions. SNRB can also be utilized to confirm a symptomatic level in patients with discordant clinical symptoms and MRI or CT myelography findings.[16,17]

CONCLUSION

There can be considerable overlap in the pain and dysfunction patterns for patients with cervical spine and shoulder pathology. However, by performing a careful history, full neurologic exam, as well as performing select provocative maneuvers, clinicians should be able to identify the etiology of pain or dysfunction. Imaging studies should be obtained only to confirm history and physical exam findings. Patients with concomitant cervical and shoulder pathology present a challenging scenario, which should be treated in a logical manner with collaboration from both treating clinicians.

REFERENCES

1. Urwin M, Symmons D, Allison T, et al. Estimating the burden of musculoskeletal disorders in the community: the comparative prevalence of symptoms at different anatomical sites, and the relation to social deprivation. Ann Rheum Dis. 1998;57(11):649-55.

2. Gatchel R. Handbook of Musculoskeletal Pain and Disability Disorders in the Workplace. New York: Springer; 2014.

3. Holmes RE, Barfield WR, Woolf SK. Clinical evaluation of nonarthritic shoulder pain: diagnosis and treatment. Phys Sportsmed. 2015:1-7.

4. Corey DL, Comeau D. Cervical radiculopathy. Med Clin North Am. 2014;98(4): 791-9, xii.

5. Binder AI. Cervical spondylosis and neck pain. BMJ. 2007;334(7592):527-31.

6. Caridi JM, Pumberger M, Hughes AP. Cervical radiculopathy: a review. HSS J. 2011;7(3):265-72.

7. Wainner RS, Gill H. Diagnosis and nonoperative management of cervical radiculopathy. J Orthop Sports Phys Ther. 2000;30(12):728-44.

8. Nordin M, Carragee EJ, Hogg-Johnson S, et al. Assessment of neck pain and its associated disorders: results of the Bone and Joint Decade 2000-2010 Task Force on Neck Pain and Its Associated Disorders. J Manipulative Physiol Ther. 2009;32(2 Suppl):S117-40.

9. Throckmorton TQ, Kraemer P, Kuhn JE, et al. Differentiating cervical spine and shoulder pathology: common disorders and key points of evaluation and treatment. Instr Course Lect. 2014;63:401-8.

10. Grimm BD, Blessinger BJ, Darden BV, et al. Mimickers of lumbar radiculopathy. J Am Acad Orthop Surg. 2015;23(1):7-17.

11. Ghasemi M, Golabchi K, Mousavi SA, et al. The value of provocative tests in diagnosis of cervical radiculopathy. J Res Med Sci. 2013;18(Suppl 1):S35-8.

12. Henderson CM, Hennessy RG, Shuey HM Jr, et al. Posterior-lateral foraminotomy as an exclusive operative technique for cervical radiculopathy: a review of 846 consecutively operated cases. Neurosurgery. 1983;13(5):504-12.

13. Pobiel RS, Schellhas KP, Eklund JA, et al. Selective cervical nerve root blockade: prospective study of immediate and longer term complications. AJNR Am J Neuroradiol. 2009;30(3):507-11.

14. Rubinstein SM, Pool JJ, van Tulder MW, et al. A systematic review of the diagnostic accuracy of provocative tests of the neck for diagnosing cervical radiculopathy. Eur Spine J. 2007;16(3):307–19.

15. Kuijper B, Tans JT, Schimsheimer RJ, et al. Degenerative cervical radiculopathy: diagnosis and conservative treatment. A review. Eur J Neurol. 2009;16(1):15-20.

16. Sasso RC, Macadaeg K, Nordmann D, et al. Selective nerve root injections can predict surgical outcome for lumbar and cervical radiculopathy: comparison to magnetic resonance imaging. J Spinal Disord Tech. 2005;18(6):471-8.

17. Eubanks JD. Cervical radiculopathy: nonoperative management of neck pain and radicular symptoms. Am Fam Physician. 2010;81(1):33-40.

18. Russell S, Triola M, Kelly P. (1995). The Precise Neurological Exam. Informatics-mednyuedu. [online] Available from https://informatics.med.nyu.edu/modules/pub/neurosurgery/index.html. [Accessed July, 2015].

19. Park MS, Kelly MP, Min WK, et al. Surgical treatment of C3 and C4 cervical radiculopathies. Spine (Phila Pa 1976). 2013;38(2):112-8.

CHAPTER 5

Groin Pain

Brett Walker, Mike Donahue

INTRODUCTION

Groin pain is a common symptom with a variety of causes and a broad differential diagnosis. Patients may commonly arrive at the orthopedic or spine surgeon's office with little or no previous workup. The surgeon must consider the whole patient, as pathology in various organ systems may produce similar symptoms. Although there are many musculoskeletal sources of groin pain, clinicians must be aware of the other causes as interventions vary widely. This chapter will explore the pertinent history, differential, physical exam and workup associated with groin pain. The focus will be orthopedic and spinal pathologies; however, other causes will be considered as well.

HISTORY

In many cases, patients will present with vague and nonspecific complaints. The patient interview should always begin with a thorough history. The "history of present illness" (HPI) should include a timeline and a chronological list of symptoms. History of trauma or inciting event is important and may help to narrow the differential diagnosis. Next, location of the pain should be recorded as specifically as possible. It may be helpful to allow the patient to draw on a diagram to provide more detail. The patient should be asked if he or she experiences any radiation of the pain. The quality, or patient description of the pain should be recorded. Pain may be described as sharp, dull, aching, burning, shooting, cramping or throbbing. Additionally, the patient should be asked if the pain is deep or superficial. Severity may be documented in several ways; many numerical or pictorial scales exist to quantify pain and may be useful in this situation. These scales are also helpful to track a patient's response to treatment in the future. Any modifying factors should also be recorded and should include any alleviating or exacerbating activities.

Particular attention should be paid to a complete review of systems. In many cases, groin pain is not found in isolation but is part of a constellation of symptoms. Careful examination of other associated complaints may help the clinician to narrow the differential. Similarly, the patient's past medical history may provide important information. Of note, past medical history should include menstrual and birth history in females. Surgical history is of particular importance. Any previous spinal, hip or abdominal surgeries should be noted. In the case of abdominal or pelvic surgery, it is important to ask whether the procedure was made with a traditional incision or using a laparoscopic technique. Older techniques for abdominal or pelvic surgery carried increased risk of nerve injury and the formation of intra-abdominal adhesions. Both of these may be potential iatrogenic causes of groin pain.

DIFFERENTIAL DIAGNOSIS

Nerve Root Compression

Lumbar Spinal Stenosis

Lumbar spinal stenosis is a common cause of pain and disability in the elderly population. Spinal stenosis refers to a narrowing of the spinal canal, which may lead to compression of the spinal cord or exiting nerve roots. Although groin pain is not a common complaint in patients with stenosis, there is a strong association between spinal foraminal stenosis, facet hypertrophy and intervertebral disk degeneration.[1] Stenosis affecting the exiting nerve roots from T12 to L2 can cause irritation of the genitofemoral, iliofemoral, ilio-inguinal and iliohypogastric nerves, leading to groin pain. Pain referral patterns from disk degeneration are well established and frequently include the groin.[2-4] Additionally, Marks demonstrated that facet joint injections from L2 to L5 reproduced groin pain.[5] Pathophysiologically, spinal stenosis slowly develops and patients commonly report an indolent course. Most often, patients complain of radicular pain and weakness of the legs. Low back pain is often reported, but this may not always be present. Patients typically report difficulty walking long distances and require frequent periods of rest. Bending forward or sitting down opens the neural foramina and decreases compression on exiting nerve roots, while extension of the lumbar spine causes increased compression. For this reason, patients with lumbar stenosis tend to prefer a flexed or "hunched" posture.

Herniated Nucleus Pulposus

Symptoms resulting from disk herniation may occur abruptly after an injury or develop slowly from degenerative disk disease. Depending on the level(s) and location of herniation, symptoms may be highly variable. Symptoms of an isolated herniated disk tend to follow more specific patterns than those

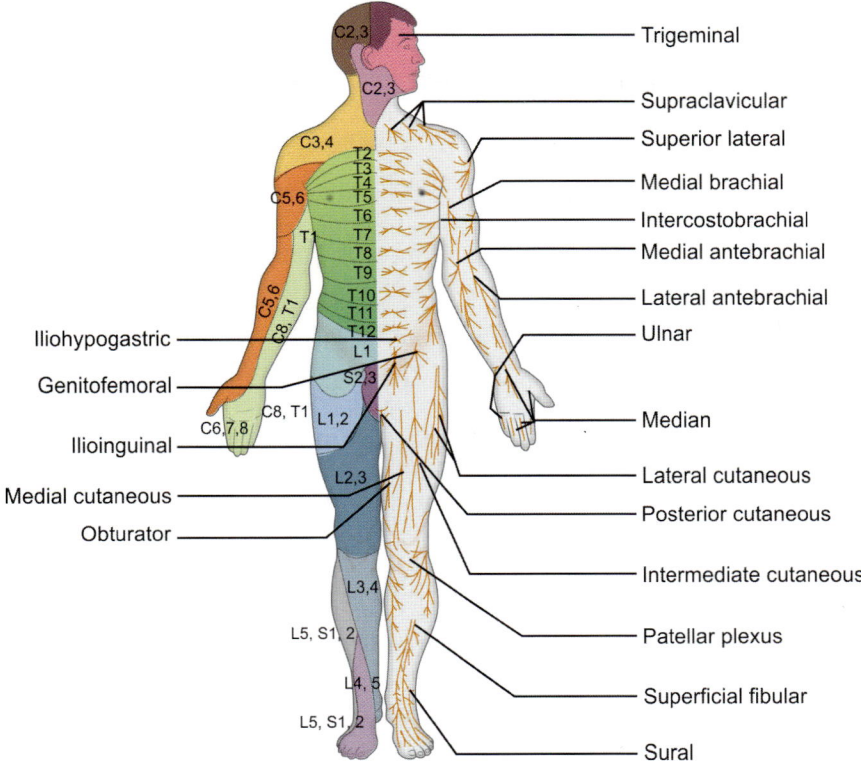

Fig. 5.1: Anterior dermatomal distributions of the nerve roots.

present with stenosis. Depending on the location of the herniation, either the traversing or exiting nerve root may be compressed. In many cases of larger herniation, both the exiting and traversing roots are compressed. Hockaday demonstrated this concept by injecting the paraspinal musculature surrounding L1 and L2, simulating pressure on the nerve roots. This is similar to conditions caused by spinal stenosis or herniation of an intervertebral disk. The patients experienced pain around the groin in the same distribution of the ilioinguinal, genitofemoral or iliohypogastric nerves.[6] Furthermore, Feinstein demonstrated that injections to L4 and L5 produced a similar pattern of pain.[7] Herniation or degeneration affecting the L1-L2 nerve roots may directly irritate the ilioinguinal, genitofemoral or iliohypogastric nerves leading to varying patterns of groin pain. Moreover, authors have reported that in addition to herniation affecting L1 and L2, a pattern of referred pain from lower lumbar herniations may also cause groin pain. Yukawa et al. retrospectively examined 512 patients with isolated lower lumbar disk herniation (L4-S1) and demonstrated that groin pain was a complaint in 4.1% of patients.[8] Figures 5.1 and 5.2 illustrate anterior and posterior dermatomal distributions of the nerve roots.

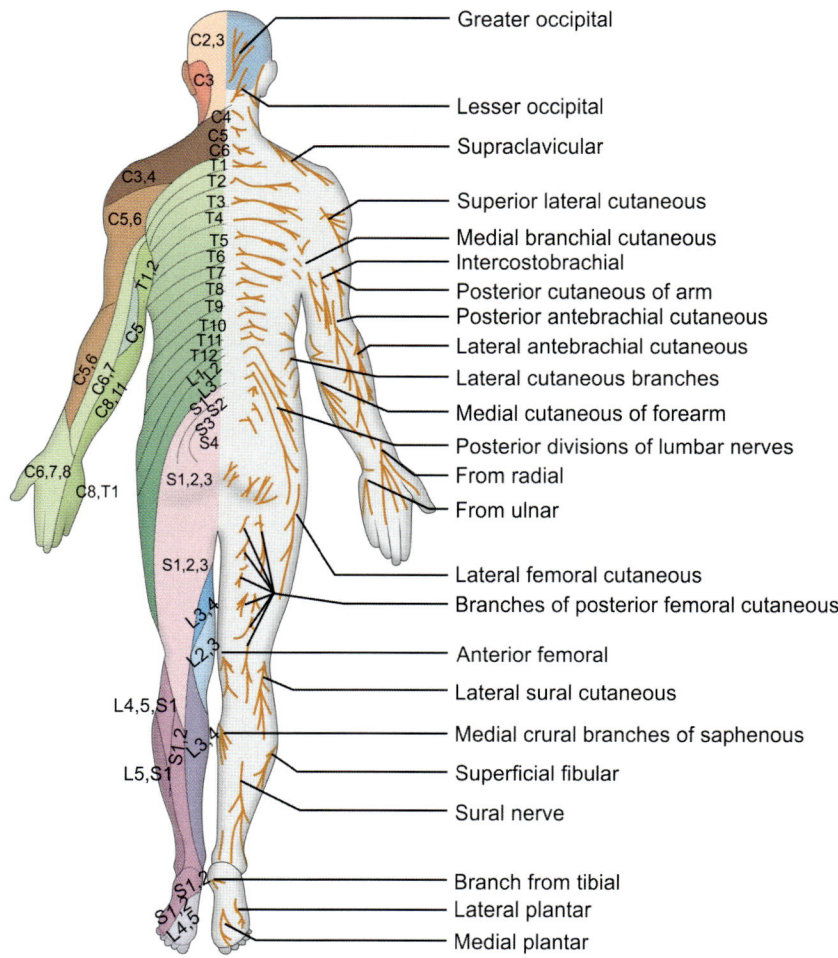

Fig. 5.2: Posterior dermatomal distributions of the nerve roots.

Peripheral Nerve Entrapment or Injury

The genitofemoral, iliohypogastric and ilioinguinal nerves provide mixed cutaneous and muscular innervation to the groin. Additionally, the lateral femoral cutaneous nerve sends sensory branches to the superior lateral thigh, which may be described as groin pain. Historically, injury or entrapment of these peripheral nerves was often iatrogenic, resulting from incisions for abdominal surgery. Procedures including hysterectomy, cesarean section, herniorrhaphy, appendectomy or abdominoplasty have been implicated in nerve injury. Since the development of laparoscopic surgery, risk of direct injury has declined; however, formation of scar tissue may still cause peripheral entrapment. Regardless of the cause, treatment remains clinically challenging. Figure 5.3 illustrates the anatomic relationship of the genitofemoral, iliohypogastric and ilioinguinal nerves.

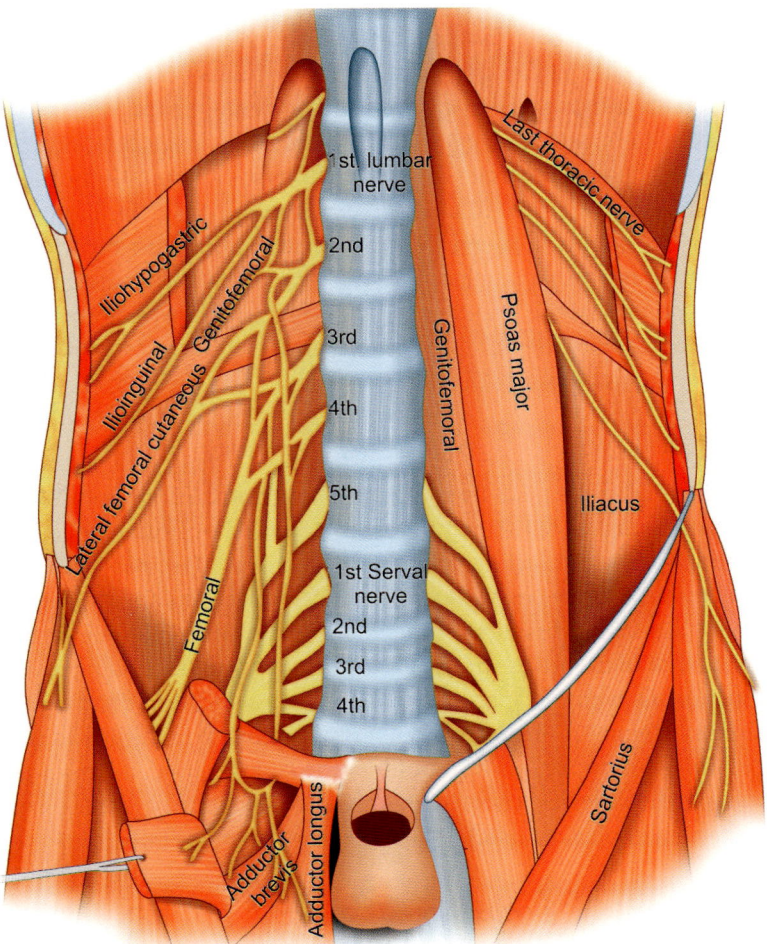

Fig. 5.3: Anatomic relationship of genitofemoral, iliohypogastric and ilioinguinal nerves.

Genitofemoral Nerve

The genitofemoral nerve arises from L1 and L2. The nerve roots coalesce within the body of the psoas muscle. The nerve exits the anterior surface of the psoas muscle at about the level of L3-L4 where it follows the fascia of the psoas muscle to the level of the ureter. It then splits into the genital and femoral branches around the inguinal ligament. The genital branch enters the inguinal canal where it innervates the skin of the scrotum and the cremaster in males or the round ligament in females. The femoral branch runs lateral to the genital branch and continues to descend posterior to the inguinal ligament and lateral to the femoral artery. It passes through the fascia lata and innervates the skin of the femoral triangle.[9]

Iliohypogastric Nerve

The iliohypogastric nerve arises from L1 with frequent T12 contribution. It contains both motor and sensory fibers. The nerve travels laterally through the psoas major muscle moving anteriorly to the quadratus lumborum. Above the iliac crest, the nerve passes through transversus abdominis muscle. About 3 cm medial to the anterior superior iliac spine (ASIS), the iliohypogastric nerve may be found between the transversus abdominis and the internal oblique muscles. The nerve splits into anterior and lateral branches, innervating the lower portion of the transverse abdominal muscle while providing cutaneous innervation to the skin just superior to the pubis and to a lesser extent, some gluteal sensation.[9]

Ilioinguinal Nerve

The ilioinguinal nerve arises from L1 with some contributions from T12 and L2. The nerve contains both motor and sensory fibers. The nerve emerges from the psoas major muscle, traveling through the anterior abdominal wall to the level of the iliac crest. The nerve passes through the transversus abdominis muscle 1 cm above the ASIS, crossing over the internal abdominal oblique muscle. The caudal half of both muscles receives innervation from the ilioinguinal nerve. It then courses with the spermatic cord in males and the round ligament of the uterus in females. The nerve innervates the pubic symphysis and either the root of the penis and anterior scrotum or the labia majora and mons pubis in the male and female, respectively.[9] Tearing of the external oblique musculature has also been implicated in injury to this nerve in contact athletes.

Lateral Femoral Cutaneous Nerve

The lateral femoral cutaneous nerve arises from L2 to L4 and is purely sensory. It courses over the iliacus muscle towards the ASIS. The nerve passes superior to the sartorius muscle where it divides into two branches. The anterior branch supplies cutaneous sensation to the lateral thigh. The posterior branch supplies cutaneous sensation to the greater trochanter and medial thigh via several smaller branches. Compression of the lateral femoral cutaneous nerve is commonly known as meralgia paresthetica.

Patients suffering from peripheral nerve entrapment or injury usually complain of burning or sharp pain in the distribution of the affected nerve which does not remit.[10] Paresthesias may also be present. The pain may be located around the medial thigh and include the penis and scrotum in males, or the labia majora and mons pubis in females. Patients may report exacerbation with movement, hip extension or Valsalva. Relief may occur with rest or hip flexion. In a case series by Viswanathan et al. the etiology was most commonly iatrogenic (herniorrhaphy, appendectomy, abdominoplasty, gynecological) with a small percentage occurring from blunt abdominal trauma.[9] In patients with a history of spinal fusion, iliac bone graft harvest may cause damage to the peripheral nerves as well. Most often, patients may be able to report a surgical or traumatic event at which time the symptoms began. This may aid in obtaining a diagnosis.

Sacroiliac Joint Dysfunction

Dysfunction of the sacroiliac (SI) joint has a highly variable presentation. In addition to lumbar or SI pain, studies have demonstrated that many patients will experience pain in the pelvis or groin. Schwarzer et al. demonstrated that groin pain was highly associated with SI joint dysfunction by utilizing diagnostic injections.[11] Similarly, Slipman and colleagues reported 14% of patients experienced groin pain with provocative SI joint injection.[12] Anatomically, the SI joint is complex consisting of bone and ligamentous structures with characteristics of both diarthrodial and synarthrodial joints.[13] History and physical examination may provide important diagnostic information implicating SI joint dysfunction. Due to the fact that the SI joints are stressed with axial load, patients will typically complain of pain which is worse while standing and alleviated with sitting. Studies on causation are limited; in 2004, Chou et al. examined the histories of patients with positive diagnostic SI joint injections. In this series, 44% of patients had a traumatic event, 21% were thought to have had a cumulative overuse injury and 35% of patients had idiopathic onset with no discernible causative event.[14] Due to the great variability in presenting symptoms, it is important for clinicians to include evaluation of the SI joints in patients complaining of groin pain. Several provocative maneuvers exist which stress the SI joint and will be discussed later in the chapter.

Hip Pathology

One of the most common causes of groin pain arises from pathology of the hip joint. Osteoarthritis, femoroacetabular impingement (FAI), avascular necrosis, labral tear and fracture all may cause patients to experience groin pain. Intra-articular pain is often described as deep pain, which is often unilateral. Suarez et al. described the "C sign", as patients will grasp their painful hip in a "C" pattern. This represents a common patient description of pain location.[15] Most causes of hip pathology develop slowly and pain has an insidious onset. In addition to pain, patients may complain of difficulty walking distances. Antalgic gait and difficulty climbing stairs or rising from a seated position may also be present with hip pathology, although a great deal of overlap exists. A thorough physical examination is important to differentiate between the many causes of intra-articular and extra-articular hip pathology and will be highlighted in this chapter.

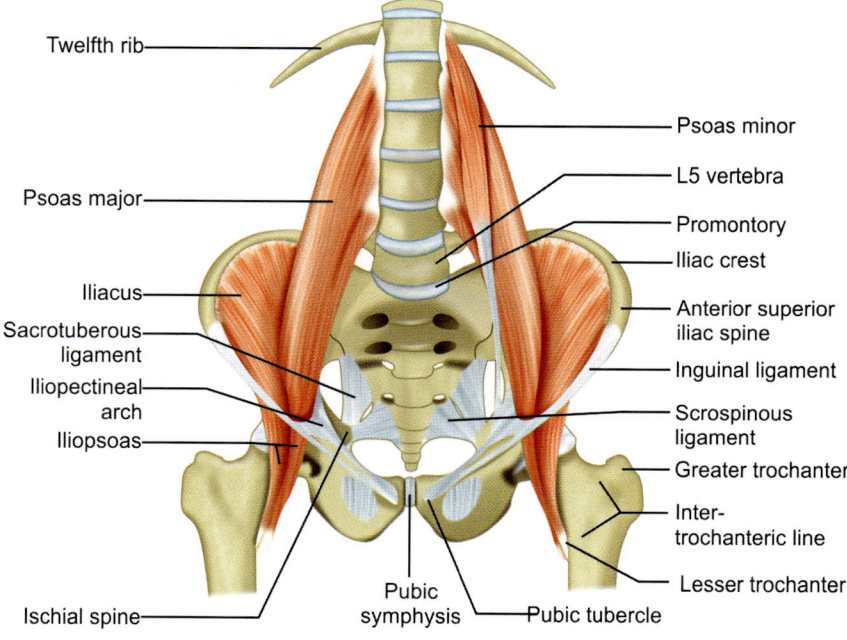

Twelfth rib

Psoas minor

L5 vertebra

Psoas major

Promontory

Iliac crest

Iliacus

Anterior superior
iliac spine

Sacrotuberous
ligament

Iliopectineal
arch

Inguinal ligament

Iliopsoas

Scrospinous
ligament

Greater trochanter

Inter-
trochanteric line

Lesser trochanter

Ischial spine

Pubic
symphysis

Pubic tubercle

Fig. 5.4: Origins and attachments of the pelvic musculature.

Tendon Injuries

Athletic injuries are becoming increasingly common in both the young and older populations. Tendon avulsions may be causes of groin pain in the athlete. Several muscles of the lower extremity have their origins on the pelvis. Figure 5.4 illustrates the attachments of the pelvic musculature. Tendinopathy or avulsion of these muscles may lead to groin or pelvic pain. The sartorius and tensor fascia latae originate at the ASIS, the rectus femoris originates at the anterior inferior iliac spine, the adductors and gracilis originate surrounding the pubic symphysis and inferior ramus, the iliopsoas attaches at the lesser trochanter of the femur and the hamstrings originate at the ischial tuberosity. The abdominal muscles also have insertions onto the iliac crest. Tenderness over any of these points with a history of athletic injury should alert the examiner to a possibility of tendinopathy or avulsion.

Athletic Pubalgia or "Sports Hernia"

Athletic pubalgia is commonly referred to as a "sports hernia". There are several theories as to the etiology of athletic pubalgia found in the literature. Some authors have suggested a weakness or tear of the posterior inguinal musculature causing occult hernia.[16] More recently, Myers et al. proposed a hyperextension injury of the pelvis causing injury to the rectus abdominis and adductor longus at or near their insertions on the pubis. In this investigation, there was no evidence of obvious or occult hernia.[17] There is no consensus whether or not this condition is more commonly found in athletes whose sport requires frequent twisting, turning or cutting motions at high speeds. However, athletes of certain sports appear to be particularly affected, including ice hockey, tennis and soccer. Diagnosis may be challenging and relies heavily on history and physical examination. Typically, patients will complain of insidious onset of unilateral groin pain, which is often described as a deep ache. The pain is aggravated by cutting and twisting activities and is alleviated by rest. Common physical examination findings include pain with resisted sit-up and hip adduction.[18] Imaging studies are typically normal, but are important to rule out other causes of groin pain. MRI will often demonstrate increased signal intensity within the affected musculotendinous structures with reactive edema of the adjacent bony anatomy. Treatment initially consists of non-surgical modalities including avoidance of strenuous activity, rest and physical therapy. For those patients whose symptoms persist after 6–8 weeks, surgical intervention may be warranted. When other causes of groin pain have been excluded, many authors have reported excellent outcomes with open or laparoscopic repair of the posterior inguinal wall.[16,19-21]

Osteitis Pubis

Osteitis pubis is described as periostitis or periosteal stress reaction of the pubic symphysis commonly observed in athletes.[22] Pain is usually described as anterior or medial often with tenderness over the pubic symphysis. Pain may radiate into the adductor musculature and may be unilateral or bilateral. Exertional activities including running, skating or cutting may aggravate symptoms while period of rest from sport usually alleviates pain.

Hernia

As previously mentioned, herniorrhaphy is a common cause of iatrogenic pelvic nerve injury. Additionally, a hernia itself may be a pain generator. There are several types of abdominal hernias that present differently. There are two types of inguinal hernias: direct and indirect. In the case of a direct inguinal hernia, the contents of the abdominal cavity protrude through a weakness in the fascia of the transversalis abdominal wall in the area of the inguinal triangle. These hernias are found medial to the inferior epigastric vessels and are not covered by the internal spermatic fascia. These hernias typically occur in adulthood. In contrast, an indirect inguinal hernia occurs through the inguinal ring, lateral to the inferior epigastric vessels where there is coverage by the internal spermatic fascia. These hernias may occur in adulthood but are often congenital. A femoral hernia is found in the femoral canal, which

Table 5.1: Potential non-orthopedic causes of groin pain.

Abdominal or pelvic adhesions	Ectopic pregnancy	Pelvic inflammatory disease
Abdominal or pelvic tumors	Endometriosis	Prostatitis
Appendicitis	Epididymitis	Testicular cancer
Bowel ischemia	Hernias	Testicular torsion
Bowel obstruction	Kidney stones	Urinary tract infection
Constipation	Lymphadenopathy	
Diverticulitis	Ovarian cysts	

allows for passage of the femoral artery and vein from the pelvis to the thigh. A paraumbilical hernia is found in the area of the umbilicus. It represents a weakness of the anterior abdominal fascia. Pain may occur if tissue becomes entrapped in the defect. In most cases of hernia, patients will complain of localized pain and upon visual inspection a prominence is noted. A Valsalva maneuver may cause an increase in size.

Other Conditions

The focus of this chapter is on the orthopedic and spinal conditions that may present with groin pain; however, it is important for the examiner to be familiar with the many other conditions that may cause these symptoms as well. Gastrointestinal, genitourinary, vascular and obstetrical conditions all may cause symptoms of groin pain and may warrant further evaluation by an appropriate specialist. Space occupying lesions including tumors are rare but must also be considered. A thorough physical examination and appropriate diagnostic testing should allow the examiner to rule in or out the possibility of these conditions. Table 5.1 lists other conditions that may present with groin pain. Table 5.2 lists possible "red flags" which may indicate more serious causes of groin pain.

PHYSICAL EXAMINATION

Visual Inspection of the Back, Abdomen and Groin

The physical examination should begin with a visual inspection. All patients should be placed into a gown, allowing for easy visualization of the skin. The clinician should visually examine the back, abdomen and groin area for any skin lesions, surgical scars, hernias or evidence of trauma.

Palpation of the Back, Abdomen and Groin

Next, the examiner should palpate the midline spine and paraspinal muscula-ture. Any areas of tenderness or step off midline should be noted. Areas of

Table 5.2: Potential "red flags" for more serious causes of groin pain.

Anorexia	Night sweats
Melena	Dysuria/polyuria
Hematochezia	Hematuria
Constitutional (fever, chills)	Pyuria
Unintended weight loss	Change in bowel or bladder habit

spasm or asymmetry of the paraspinal musculature should be diagrammed. Next, the abdomen and groin should be palpated. If an umbilical, femoral or inguinal hernia is noted the examiner may palpate to determine if they can recreate the patient's pain. The examiner may attempt to reduce the hernia by applying direct pressure. Hernias which are not able to be reduced and those which are symptomatic may require more acute intervention. Any surgical scars in the abdomen or groin should be palpated as well. Formation of scar tissue and adhesions may cause pain in the groin. The examiner should also palpate along the paths of the ilioinguinal, genitofemoral and iliohypogastric nerves. Any pain along the course of these nerves may indicate peripheral nerve compression.

Observation of Gait and Posture

Visual gait analysis may provide insight to associated conditions or syndromes. An antalgic gait may be observed when a patient experiences pain with ambulation and may be a sign of hip joint pathology. A Trendelenburg gait results from hip abductor weakness, which could represent weakness to L5 or be iatrogenic from previous hip surgery. Posture may also provide important diagnostic clues. A patient who stands with a "hunched" or forward bent posture may be suffering from lumbar stenosis.

Lumbar Range of Motion

The patient should be taken through range of motion of the lumbar spine. Flexion, extension, lateral bending and rotation should be recorded. Exacerbation of the patient's symptoms with any of these motions should also be noted. Patients suffering from spinal stenosis or herniated disk may experience exacerbation of their symptoms with extension and flexion, respectively.

Neurologic Examination (Motor, Sensory, Reflexes)

A thorough neurological examination of the lower extremities should be completed bilaterally. Any asymmetry in strength, sensation or reflexes should be noted. A list of relevant reflexes is listed in Table 5.3.

Table 5.3: Relevant cervical, lumbar and sacral nerve testing.

Spinal level	Muscles tested	Reflex
C5	Deltoid, biceps	Biceps
C6	Brachioradialis, wrist extensors	Brachioradialis
C7	Triceps, wrist flexors	Triceps
C8	Middle, index finger flexion	–
L3	Hip flexors, adductors, knee extensors	–
L4	Knee extensors, ankle dorsiflexors	Patellar
L5	Extensor hallucis longus	–
S1	Ankle plantar flexors	Achilles

Table 5.4: Normal hip range of motion.

Position	Normal range of motion (degrees)
Flexion	125
Extension	10–15
Internal rotation	40
External rotation	45
Abduction	45
Adduction	30

Hip Range of Motion/Log Roll

A thorough physical examination of the patient's hips is important in the evaluation of groin pain. Hip range of motion (flexion, extension, internal rotation, external rotation, abduction and adduction) should be tested and documented bilaterally. Normal range of motions can be found in Table 5.4. Decreased range of motion may be found in a variety of pathologies including osteoarthritis, FAI or even fracture. A log roll may be useful for evaluating possible occult femoral neck fractures. With the patient lying supine on the examination table, the hip and knee are extended. Next, the examiner will "roll" the leg from internal rotation and external rotation. A positive test will produce pain in the groin and necessitate further testing.

Heel Strike

Heel strike may also be a useful test for occult femoral neck fracture. While the patient is lying supine, the examiner will strike the patient's heel providing an axial force on the leg. Pain in the groin with this technique represents a positive result, and may indicate occult or stress fracture.

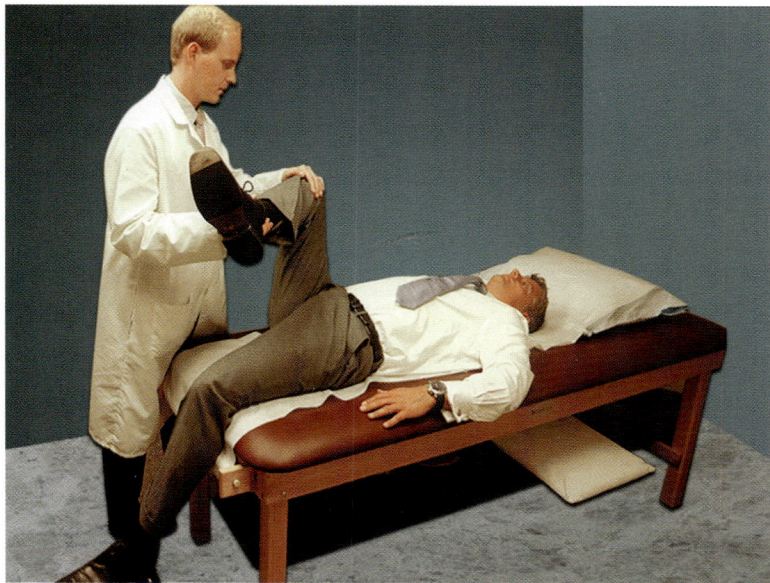

Fig. 5.5: The external rotatory impingement test. (With the patient supine, and the hip and knee flexed to 90°, the examiner provides external rotation and abduction to the hip joint.)

External or Internal Rotatory Impingement

With the hip and knee flexed to 90°, the examiner provides adduction and internal rotation followed by abduction and external rotation forces through the hip joint. It is important to evaluate the patient with the non-affected leg flexed to 90/90 as well to eliminate any pelvic tilt. A positive test will reproduce the patient's pain and may indicate FAI or other intra-articular pathology. The external and internal rotatory impingement tests are illustrated in Figures 5.5 and 5.6, respectively.

Testing of the Sacroiliac Joint

The SI joint may be examined by performing several provocative maneuvers. For each of the listed examinations, a positive result is indicated by repro-duction of the patient's pain.

FABER Test

Stresses the SI joint by placing the supine patient's hip in the flexed, abducted, externally rotated and extended position. Pain around the area of the ipsilateral SI joint is considered a positive finding; however, there may be significant overlap with hip pathology. The Flexion, ABduction, and External Rotation (FABER) test is demonstrated in Figure 5.7.

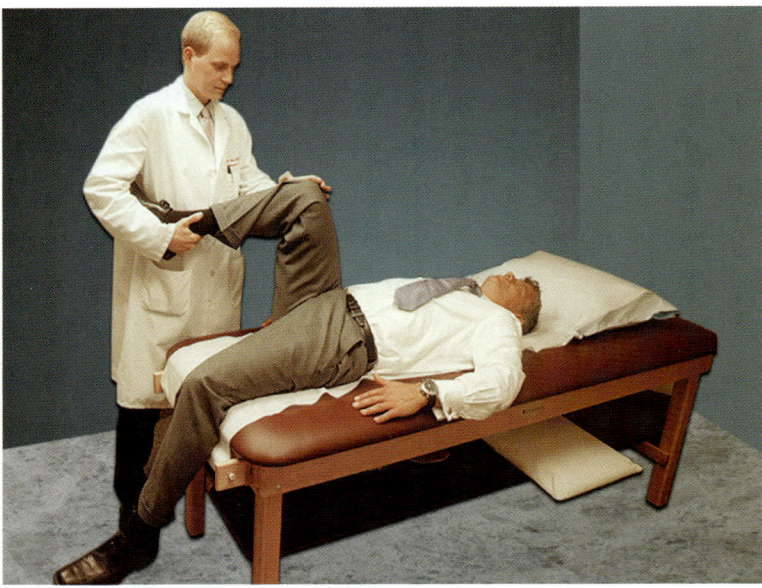

Fig. 5.6: The internal rotatory impingement test. (With the patient supine, and the hip and knee flexed to 90°, the examiner provides internal rotation and adduction to the hip joint.)

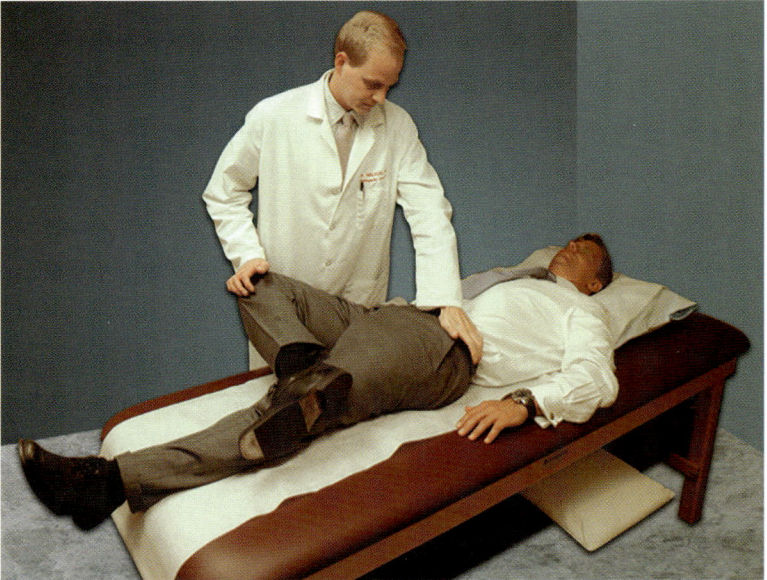

Fig. 5.7: The Flexion, ABduction, and External Rotation (FABER) test. (With the patient supine, the patient's knee is placed into the "figure 4" position as shown. Downward force is applied to the knee by the examiner. The examiner's opposite hand is used to apply counter-pressure to the contralateral anterior superior iliac spine (ASIS).)

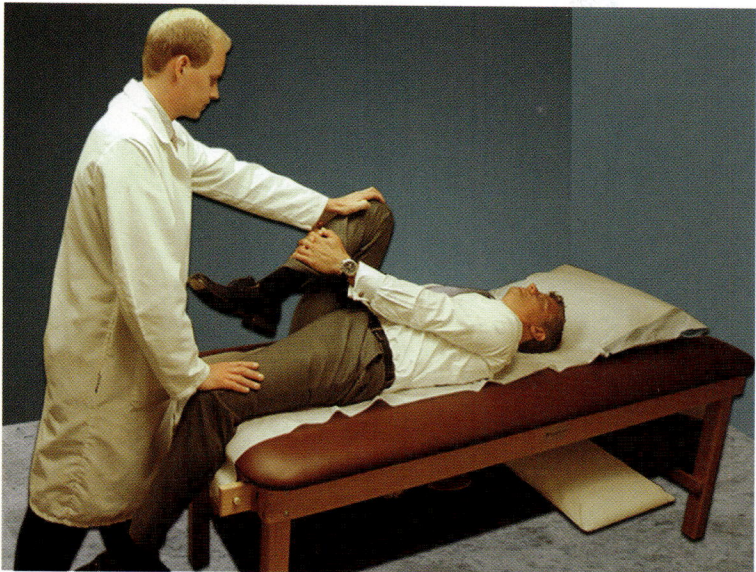

Fig. 5.8: The Gaenslen's test. (With the patient holding his or her hip and knee in a flexed position, the contralateral leg is left to suspend off of the examination table. The examiner applies a flexion force to the hip and knee while the opposite hand maintains contralateral hip extension.)

Gaenslen's Test

Places torsional stress across the SI joint. While lying supine, the patient's asymptomatic hip and knee is flexed to the abdomen while allowing the contralateral leg to hang from the table. Force is applied to both legs; the flexed knee is further flexed by the examiner while a downward force is directed to the hanging leg (symptomatic side). Pain in the area of the SI joints is considered a positive finding. Gaenslen's test is demonstrated in Figure 5.8.

Iliac Gapping and Compression Testing

The iliac gapping test provides a distraction force to the anterior ligaments of the SI joints. With the patient lying supine, the examiner applies a downward force onto both anterior superior iliac spines. This is shown in Figure 5.9.

The iliac compression test is performed with the patient in the lateral decubitus position. The examiner provides a downward force through the iliac wing which translates to a compressive force through the SI joints.

Single Leg Standing

While supporting the patient's hands to avoid falls, the patient is asked to stand on one leg. This position will place a sheer stress across the SI joint of the planted leg.

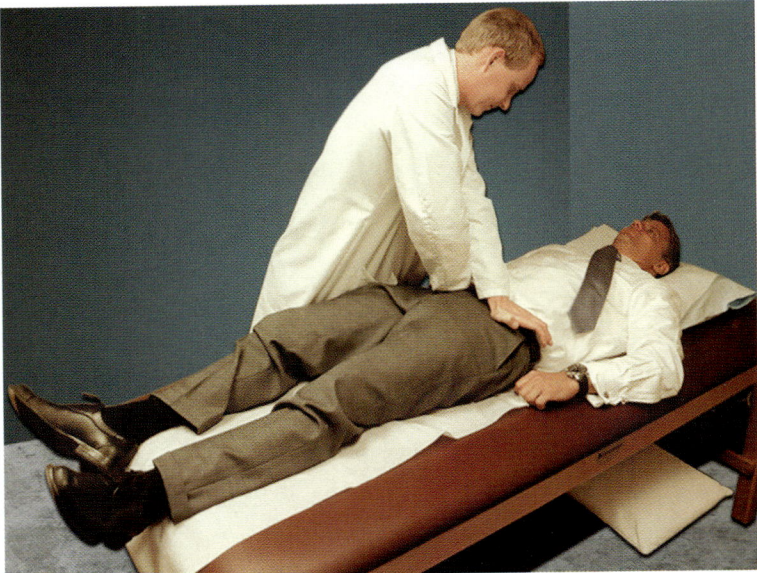

Fig. 5.9: Iliac gapping test. (With the patient supine, the examiner crosses his or her arms and applies a downward force to each anterior superior iliac spine (ASIS). This creates anterior gapping and posterior compression.)

Pubic Symphysis Examination

While the patient is supine, the examiner should directly palpate over the anterior pubic symphysis. Pain with palpation should be recorded. The examiner may provide stress across the pubic symphysis by having the patient perform resisted adduction of the legs at 0°, 20°, 40° and 60° of hip flexion. Additionally, single leg squatting or hopping may also produce pain by irritating the bone or periosteum of the pubic symphysis.

IMAGING STUDIES

X-Ray

Plain radiography should be the first line imaging study performed, especially in the presence of trauma. X-rays of the pelvis, hips and lumbar spine should be obtained on the patient complaining of groin pain. In addition to fracture, plain radiography may be helpful in screening for osteoarthritis of the hips or spine, skeletal tumors, avulsions and stress reactions.

Computed Tomography

Computed tomography (CT) examination provides excellent visualization of skeletal anatomy and pathology. Images are reconstructed in multiple planes and can be manipulated. Additionally, contrast may be administered which can provide additional diagnostic information. A drawback of CT scanning, however, is the high radiation dose.

Magnetic Resonance Imaging

Magnetic resonance imaging (MRI) is a valuable tool for the diagnosis of soft tissue pathology that is not well visualized on CT or X-ray. It is also especially useful in evaluating edema; both in the soft tissues and bone. In addition to its diagnostic value for spinal conditions, many other orthopedic conditions may be diagnosed with MRI. Muscular or myotendinous injury is visualized well using MRI. Findings include increased fluid signal on T2-weighted images within the tendon, as well as focal bone marrow edema at the attachment site of the muscle. Osteitis pubis represents a stress reaction of the pubic symphysis. MRI evaluation demonstrates bone marrow edema which is often bilateral and diffuse.[23] Stress fractures may be missed on plain radiography. MRI detects bone marrow edema in the area of stress reaction and is useful to make a diagnosis. Pathologies of the hips are also well evaluated with MRI. Labral pathologies are well visualized. Evaluation of the abdominal soft tissues also allows for evaluation of hernias.

Ultrasound

Ultrasound has emerged as a useful tool for the diagnosis of many musculo-skeletal pathologies. It has the benefits of being inexpensive, able to be quickly performed and is widely available. Ultrasound provides a real time, dynamic examination which allows the examiner to evaluate tissue during motion. Newer technology has made the availability of ultrasound in the orthopedic clinic possible; however, there is a learning curve and reliability is often user dependent. A skilled sonographer may evaluate tendinopathies, hematomas, muscle injuries, the hip joint, effusions and hernias. In the case of hernia, the dynamic nature of the examination is helpful for surgical planning. Reducible hernias may not require surgical intervention, while those that are irreducible or show signs of bowel incarceration require more immediate attention.

Table 5.5 summarizes imaging modalities.

FURTHER DIAGNOSTIC STUDIES

Electromyelography

Electromyelography (EMG) tests the conduction velocities of electrical signals of nerves. Most commonly, it is used to test the nerves of the extremities.

Table 5.5: Imaging studies summarized.

Study	Pathologies visualized
X-ray	Fracture, tendon avulsions, FAI
CT	Fracture, intra-articular loose bodies, FAI
MRI	Occult fracture, avascular necrosis, labral injury, chondral injury, tendinopathy, muscle injury, osteitis pubis, hernia, degenerative disk disease, nerve root compression, peripheral nerve compression
Ultrasound	Hernia, tendinopathy, myopathy, peripheral nerve compression, some evaluation of the hip joint, evaluation of the ovaries and testicles

(CT: Computed tomography; MRI: Magnetic resonance imaging; FAI: Femoroacetabular impingement).

By using these same principles, an examiner may also test the ilioinguinal, iliofemoral, genitofemoral and iliohypogastric nerves. Abnormalities of conduction velocities may provide information leading to a diagnosis of nerve entrapment.

Anesthesia Injection

Injection of local anesthetic into an area of nerve entrapment may provide important diagnostic information. The goal of the injection is to provide temporary relief of nerve pain related to entrapment. If the injection successfully provides relief, the examiner may be confident of the diagnosis of peripheral nerve entrapment. This technique may also be used to evaluate the SI joints. Injection of analgesic medication into the joint may provide symptomatic relief when the patient's symptoms are due to SI dysfunction.

CONCLUSION

Patients complaining of groin pain pose a difficult challenge to clinicians. A wide range of pathologies involving many organ systems may present with similar symptoms. A detailed history, complete physical exam and appropriate imaging studies are critical to obtaining a proper diagnosis. Although many causes of groin pain are musculoskeletal, it is important for surgeons to recognize potential "red flags" which may indicate more serious etiologies.

REFERENCES

1. Splendiani A, Ferrari F, Barile A, et al. Occult neural foraminal stenosis caused by association between disc degeneration and facet joint osteoarthritis: demonstration with dedicated upright MRI system. Radiol Med. 2014;119(3):164-74.
2. Oikawa Y, Ohtori S, Koshi T, et al. Lumbar disc degeneration induces persistent groin pain. Spine. 2012;37(2):114-8.

3. Sameda H, Takahashi Y, Takahashi K, et al. Dorsal root ganglion neurones with dichotomising afferent fibres to both the lumbar disc and the groin skin. A possible neuronal mechanism underlying referred groin pain in lower lumbar disc diseases. J Bone Joint Surg Br. 2003;85(4):600-3.

4. Takahashi Y, Sato A, Nakamura SI, et al. Regional correspondence between the ventral portion of the lumbar intervertebral disc and the groin mediated by a spinal reflex. A possible basis of discogenic referred pain. Spine. 1998;23(17):1853-8; discussion 9.

5. Marks R. Distribution of pain provoked from lumbar facet joints and related structures during diagnostic spinal infiltration. Pain. 1989;39(1):37-40.

6. Hockaday JM, Whitty CW. Patterns of referred pain in the normal subject. Brain. 1967;90(3):481-96.

7. Feinstein B, Langton JN, Jameson RM, et al. Experiments on pain referred from deep somatic tissues. J Bone Joint Surg Am. 1954;36-A(5):981-97.

8. Yukawa Y, Kato F, Kajino G, et al. Groin pain associated with lower lumbar disc herniation. Spine (Phila Pa 1976). 1997;22(15):1736-9; discussion 1740.

9. Viswanathan A, Kim DH, Reid N, et al. Surgical management of the pelvic plexus and lower abdominal nerves. Neurosurgery. 2009;65(4 Suppl):A44-51.

10. Rassner L. Lumbar plexus nerve entrapment syndromes as a cause of groin pain in athletes. Curr Sports Med Rep. 2011;10(2):115-20.

11. Schwarzer AC, Aprill CN, Bogduk N. The sacroiliac joint in chronic low back pain. Spine. 1995;20(1):31-7.

12. Slipman CW, Jackson HB, Lipetz JS, et al. Sacroiliac joint pain referral zones. Arch Phys Med Rehabil. 2000;81(3):334-8.

13. Vleeming A, Schuenke MD, Masi AT, et al. The sacroiliac joint: an overview of its anatomy, function and potential clinical implications. J Anat. 2012; 221(6):537-67.

14. Chou LH, Slipman CW, Bhagia SM, et al. Inciting events initiating injection-proven sacroiliac joint syndrome. Pain Med. 2004;5(1):26-32.

15. Suarez JC, Ely EE, Mutnal AB, et al. Comprehensive approach to the evaluation of groin pain. J Am Acad Orthop Surg. 2013;21(9):558-70.

16. Hackney RG. The sports hernia: a cause of chronic groin pain. Br J Sports Med. 1993;27(1):58-62.

17. Meyers WC, Foley DP, Garrett WE, et al. Management of severe lower abdominal or inguinal pain in high-performance athletes. PAIN (Performing Athletes with Abdominal or Inguinal Neuromuscular Pain Study Group). Am J Sports Med. 2000;28(1):2-8.

18. Farber AJ, Wilckens JH. Sports hernia: diagnosis and therapeutic approach. J Am Acad Orthop Surg. 2007;15(8):507-14.

19. Susmallian S, Ezri T, Elis M, et al. Laparoscopic repair of "sportsman's hernia" in soccer players as treatment of chronic inguinal pain. Med Sci Monit. 2004;10(2):Cr52-4.

20. Steele P, Annear P, Grove JR. Surgery for posterior inguinal wall deficiency in athletes. J Sci Med Sport. 2004;7(4):415-21; discussion 422-3.

21. Malycha P, Lovell G. Inguinal surgery in athletes with chronic groin pain: the 'sportsman's' hernia. Aust N Z J Surg. 1992;62(2):123-5.

22. Hiti CJ, Stevens KJ, Jamati MK, et al. Athletic osteitis pubis. Sports Med. 2011;41(5):361-76.

23. Khan W, Zoga AC, Meyers WC. Magnetic resonance imaging of athletic pubalgia and the sports hernia: current understanding and practice. Magn Reson Imaging Clin N Am. 2013;21(1):97-110.

CHAPTER 6

Leg Pain/Weakness/Numbness

Andrew G Park, Karim Shafi, Tristan Fried, Alexander R Vaccaro

INTRODUCTION

The art of medicine lies in establishing a diagnosis related to a patient problem, so that a treatment may be implemented. Often this process is difficult, labor intensive for both the patient and physician, and expensive. However these challenges can be mitigated if a concrete differential diagnosis can be generated. In medicine a differential diagnosis is the distinguishing of a particular disease or condition from others presenting with similar signs and symptoms.[1] This process is especially important with a chief complaint of leg pain, weakness, and numbness given the almost limitless possible pathologies. While there is no one particular strategy that has been proven to be superior, the following will present a general frame of reference to guide care givers in working up the particular problem of leg pain, weakness, and/ or numbness. Following a general discussion will be a systems or problem based approach to diagnosis.

HISTORY

The physician encounter begins with history taking. A complete history entails the age and gender of the patient, history of present illness (HPI), past medical history (PMH), past surgical history (PSH), social history (SH), medications, allergies, and any treatments previously tried in relation to leg pain. The pneumonic "COLDER AS" can help guide the history and refers to character, onset, location, duration, exacerbation, remitting factors, associated symptoms, and severity. From a spine surgeon's perspective it is important to note the chronology and progression of symptoms, bowel or bladder difficulties, balance problems resulting in falls, and difficulty with fine motor tasks of the hands. These particular questions help to not overlook cervical and thoracic spine pathology such as myelopathy and other forms of spinal cord compression, which may present with predominantly lower extremity symptoms. In addition, questions about specific treatments and their effect as they pertain to the spine should include but are not limited to: systemic steroid and non-steroidal anti-inflammatory drug (NSAID) administration, chiropractic medicine, acupuncture, epidural or transforaminal spine injections, physical therapy, bracing, and traction therapy.

PHYSICAL

From the perspective of a spine surgeon every patient should undergo a complete spine exam. Depending on the presenting complaints further examination of vascular, musculoskeletal, neurologic, integumentary, and/or abdominal systems may be indicated. Details of specific provocative tests will be presented along with the relevant clinical problem.

Musculoskeletal issues may present with a history of a chronic or acute injury. It is important to perform a physical exam looking at strength, range of motion, and tenderness. Generally in isolated musculoskeletal leg injuries such as muscular and ligament strains, sensation of the dermatomes and peripheral pulses will be normal. Leg overuse injuries such as arthritis or bursitis can be present in the hip, knee, or ankle joints, commonly with joint line tenderness. Bursitis results from inflammation of the fluid filled sacs that buffers bony prominences from surrounding soft tissues. Weakness may be present due to pain inhibition; however there will be no sensory changes.[2]

DIFFERENTIAL DIAGNOSES

When determining a differential diagnosis, start with the chief complaint and look for key symptoms to narrow the diagnosis from the most common to rare conditions. The remaining sections will detail system or problem specific groupings. A common pneumonic, "$VI^2N^2D^2ICA^3T^2E$," will be used for a systematic approach to diagnosis: Vascular, inflammatory & infectious, neoplastic & neurologic, degenerative & deficiency, idiopathic, congenital, autoimmune & allergic & anatomic, trauma & toxins, endocrine.

VASCULAR

Peripheral Vascular Disease: Vascular Claudication: The presence of diminished or absent peripheral pulses often indicates peripheral vascular disease. Attention to the skin is important to look for changes in color, hairlessness, atrophic changes, or shiny skin. Symptoms of vascular claudication are frequently described as a constant ache or burning sensation in the lower extremity often relieved by rest. If the legs develop ulcers, weeping, or gangrene this may indicate severe vascular occlusion that needs to be addressed by a peripheral vascular surgeon.

Deep Vein Thrombosis: Deep venous thrombosis is a less likely diagnosis for patients presenting with acute leg pain, however should always be considered because of the serious implications if missed. Typical presentation is calf swelling and pain, which may be worse with palpation. Risk factors include immobility, obesity, pregnancy, malignancy, prior thrombosis, and recent surgery. Repeat and chronic deep venous thrombosis can stretch the venous valves leading to vascular incompetence and varicose veins. Frequently a deep venous thrombosis presents as unilateral leg edema and erythema. The physical exam is notoriously unreliable for this potentially serious condition. There may be a palpable cord that is appreciated in the posterior calf or thigh. Homan's sign, calf pain upon passive ankle dorsiflexion, may be positive.

INFECTION

Superficial Soft Tissue Infection/Abscess: Skin and soft tissue infections (SSTIs) often involve a gradual onset of diffuse symptoms such as fever and general discomfort. Physical exam demonstrates warmth, edema, and pain in the affected area. Palpable fluid that can be moved in waves may indicate presence of an abscess. This collection helps differentiate an abscess from other forms of infection, such as cellulitis. A deeper infection of the psoas muscle, an iliopsoas abscess, presents with pain to the hip, thigh, and groin area, due to innervation of the L2-L4 nerve roots. Patients may present with limp, fever, and back pain, and an ultrasound may be helpful in making a diagnosis.[3] A history of previous surgeries or open wounds should raise suspicion of possible routes of infection. MRI can be used to confirm initial clinical diagnosis of superficial musculoskeletal infection and can determine the extent of infection.[4]

Cellulitis: Patients with lower limb cellulitis often exhibit systemic and/or dermatologic symptoms. Common findings of systemic infection or inflammatory processes include fever, tachycardia, and hypotension.[5] Capillary dilation contributes to the classic finding of a spreading reddening of the skin that persists with elevation of the leg and is accompanied by heat, edema, and pain to touch. The skin may also take on the appearance of an orange peel.[5] Importantly, cellulitis should be used to describe a superficial infection that does not present with a collection of fluid. Lab studies may demonstrate non-specific findings such as increased WBC count, C-reactive protein, and sedimentation rate but may not be necessary to confirm a diagnosis in most cases.

Septic Joint: Risk factors for septic arthritis include osteoarthritis, prosthetic joints, or recent joint trauma. Pain, swelling, erythema and a diminished range of motion in the presence of one or more risk factors may indicate septic arthritis. Diagnostic tests should include gross examination of aspirated synovial fluid. Gram-stain smears and microbe cultures are extremely reliable tests in indicating the presence of a septic joint. MRI studies provide evidence of changes in soft tissue such as presence of joint capsule distension, local fluid build-up, and a "fat pad" sign. These findings support the diagnosis of septic arthritis.[6]

INFLAMMATORY

Rheumatoid Arthritis: Early stages of rheumatoid arthritis often present with indistinct symptoms, including inflammatory polyarthritis and morning stiffness. As the disease progresses, patients experience more characteristic symptoms of RA, developing joint erosions and rheumatoid nodules as the synovial membranes become thickened. Patients often describe difficulties performing activities of daily living (ADLs), such as walking, climbing stairs, opening jars or doors, or performing their normal job. Morning stiffness is often described in peripheral joints lasting longer than 30 minutes, with symptoms lasting longer than 6 weeks. Serologic testing for elevated rheumatoid factor (RF) and anti-Cyclic Citrullinated Peptide (CCP) antibodies are indicated, although RF may also be elevated in healthy patients.[7]

Gout: The initial presentation of gout involves recurrent inflammatory arthritis. The classical case involves the metatarsophalangeal joint of the big toe, where patients describe a hot, biting pain. Diagnostic testing should be performed to rule out other causes of arthritic pain, including pseudogout or rheumatoid arthritis. Synovial fluid sampling via arthrocentesis reveals characteristic monosodium urate crystals. Further lab tests of fluid samples should be performed to rule out septic joint. The presence of tophi also suggests gouty arthritis as opposed to other causes of inflammatory pain.[8]

NEOPLASTIC

Primary Bone/Soft Tissue Tumor: Benign osteomas are variable in their clinical presentation, and symptoms depend on location. Radiographs may demonstrate dense, white masses with clearly delineated borders.[9] A biopsy is also indicated as histological data can be used to differentiate between types of bone tumors.[9] Histologic studies may reveal mature bone with decreased marrow, and lamella may have the appearance of cancellous or compact bone.

NEUROLOGIC

Neurologic causes of leg pain are among the most common reason for presentation to the spine clinician. These can be caused by compression of the neural elements in the lower back, or less commonly from peripheral neuropathies.

Peripheral Neuropathies: Initial presentations of peripheral neuropathy include either positive sensory symptoms, such as pain or paresthesia, or negative symptoms, such as numbness or loss of proprioception. Physical exam may show decreased/absent muscle stretch reflexes or decreased/absent perception of general, proprioceptive, and pain sensations, including light touch, temperature, and pinprick test. Any distribution of loss of sensation may help localize the lesion to specific nerve roots based on dermatomal distribution. Distal lower limb weakness may be present, and patients with more advanced stages of neuropathy may demonstrate foot drop or have a history of ankle sprains due to weakness and altered gait. Weakness of axial muscles is less common in neuropathies. Inspection and palpation of the lower limb can be used to determine presence of atrophy and measure muscle tone, which is generally decreased. Increased tone suggests the presence of an upper motor neuron lesion.[10]

Peripheral Nerve Entrapment: One cause of sensory or motor loss is due to compression of peripheral nerves throughout the lower extremity. Mild nerve entrapment results in reversible ischemia causing transient symptoms, while chronic compression may lead to demyelination and more severe, lasting effects.[10] Table 6.1 summarizes common sites of peripheral nerve entrapment and their effects.

Table 6.1: Common sites of peripheral nerve entrapments and their effects.

Nerve	Spinal root(s)	Sensory effects	Motor effects
Ilioinguinal	• L1	• Hyperesthesia • Pain along ilioinguinal ligament, inner thigh, medial groin • Pain with Hip Hyperextension	• NA
Obturator [11]	• L2, L3, L4	• Pain along medial thigh	• Weakness with hip adduction • Some wasting of muscles of medial thigh (adductor longus, adductor brevis, gracilis)
Lateral femoral cutaneous	• L2, L3	• Burning pain and/or parasthesia in lateral thigh • Symptoms exacerbated by tight belts, walking, standing • Pain relief with hip flexion	• NA
Sciatic [12,13]	• L4, L5, S1, S2, S3	• Pain and/or parasthesia along hip and gluteal region • Pain exacerbated with knee extension	• Characteristic limp to relieve pain
Saphenous [14]	• L3, L4	• Pain along anterior and deep thigh, knee, medial aspect of leg, medial malleolus	• NA

Contd…

Contd...

Nerve	Spinal root(s)	Sensory effects	Motor effects
Common peroneal [15]	• L4, L5, S1, S2	• Paraesthesia, diminished sensation over lateral leg, dorsal foot	• Decreased ankle dorsiflexion ("Foot Drop") • Steppage Gait
Superficial peroneal [16]	• L4, L5, S1	• Pain and/or paresthesia along dorsal foot • Pain exacerbated with increased activity, inversion, plantar flexion (stretches nerve)	• Weakness with eversion of foot • Possible atrophy of lateral aspect of leg (peroneus longus, peroneus brevis)
Deep peroneal [17]	• L4, L5	• Pain and/or parasthesia along dorsal foot • Pain may begin in first dorsal webspace • Tinel sign along nerve pathway	• Weakness with foot dorsiflexion • Weakness and/or atrophy of extensor digitorum brevis • Possible edema of tibialis anterior
Posterior Tibial [18]	• L4, L5, S1, S2, S3	• Pain and/or parasthesia along heel, plantar foot • Hyperasthesia • Pain exacerbated with increased activity and is worse at night • Some pain relief when shoes removed	• Weakened ankle and toe plantar flexion • Possible atrophy of intrinsic muscles of foot
Lateral Plantar [18]	• L4, L5, S1, S2, S3	• Pain and or/parasthesia along lateral aspect of plantar foot (fifth toe and half of fourth toe)	• Weakness of intrinsic muscles of foot • Possible atrophy of intrinsic muscles of the foot
Sural [19]	• L4, L5, S1, S2, S3, S4	• Pain along posterolateral leg, lateral aspect of foot and fifth toe • Pain worse overnight and exacerbated by exercise/increased activity	• NA

Charcot Marie Tooth: Charcot Marie Tooth (CMT) disease is a common hereditary disorder that leads to length-dependent axonal degradation. CMT presents with loss of sensation along dermatomes and atrophy along extremities. The classic presentation involves weakness and muscle loss (atrophy) of the distal leg accompanied by loss of sensation and absent reflexes. Patients also often describe moderate to severe, symmetric neuropathic pain. CMT associated pain may include cramps and paresthesia and responds poorly to treatment with either non-steroidal anti-inflammatory drugs (NSAIDs) or opiates. This pain stems from various pathological processes, which include dorsal root ganglion, spinal root, and CNS-associated demyelination and axon degradation. Nerve conduction studies also demonstrate uniformly slowed nerve conduction velocities, which helps differentiate this disorder from acquired peripheral polyneuropathies.[20]

TIA/Stroke (Thalamic): Stroke is defined as a decrease in blood supply to the brain, causing cerebral hypoxia when blood flow falls below 18–20 ml/100 g tissue/min.[10] Strokes are classified as either ischemic or hemorrhagic. A transient ischemic attack (TIA) involves rapid reversal of ischemia, with symptoms only lasting a few minutes to hours. Stroke symptoms are characterized by sudden onset of neurologic deficits, including hemiparesis, hemiplegia, facial droop, visual field defects, paresthesia, and aphasia. Lower limb weakness may occur as a result of anterior cerebral artery ischemia, affecting the side contralateral to the lesion. Infarcts of the ventroposterolateral (VPL) nucleus of the thalamus may induce Thalamic Pain Syndrome.[10] Pain is described as "burning" or "shooting" and may be exacerbated by light touch stimuli. Affected areas include the face, arm, trunk, and leg ispilateral to the lesion.[21] Clinical diagnostic tests include the FAST (Face Arm Speech Test), which looks for facial palsy, upper limb weakness, and aphasia, and ROSIER (Recognition of Stroke in the Emergency Room) scale, a more thorough test which can differentiate between strokes and their mimics.[22] Imaging studies include CT (computed tomography) scan, while MRI data can detect and characterize ischemic strokes. Blood vessel evaluation includes MR angiography (MRA) and CT angiography (CTA) studies, which show any stenosis of intracranial vessels.[23]

Multiple Sclerosis: Leg pain associated with multiple sclerosis is not uncommon, and often presents in more than one limb. Neuropathic pain may be continuous or intermittent and is described as burning or feelings of strong pressure. Patients may also experience acute bouts of generalized dysesthesia.[24] Diagnosis of MS is based on positive findings upon clinical exam, including weakness, paresthesia, vision loss, or internuclear opthalmoplegia (INO).[10] Symptoms are diffuse, and, unfortunately, there are none that are pathognomonic to MS. Evidence of neurologic disturbances and a history of previous episodes are used to make an accurate diagnosis. MRI studies can be used if clinical evidence is insufficient. Images demonstrate multiple brain and/or spinal cord lesions, and specific criteria have been established in diagnosing MS.[25]

Amyotrophic Lateral Sclerosis: Amyotrophic lateral sclerosis (ALS) typically presents with both upper and lower motor neuron signs. The latter include progressive muscle wasting and fasiculations. Patients also exhibit progressive weakness, beginning distally in the hands, feet, and legs. Upper motor neuron signs include hyper-reflexive tendons and clonus.[10,26]

Babinski's sign, splaying of the toes and extension upon sharp touch along the sole of the foot, and Hoffman's sign, flexion of first distal phalange when flicking third distal phalange, may be present. Diagnosis is based on the combination of upper and lower motor signs upon clinical exam, which distinguishes ALS from other neurological disorders.

DEGENERATIVE

Hip, Knee, Ankle Arthritis: The diagnosis of arthritis includes symptoms such as pain, swelling, and decreased range of motion. The time course is chronic with progressively worsening symptoms. Examination usually reveals pain with decreased range of motion and crepitus. The clinician should observe the patient walk to assess for an antalgic gait. The FABER (flexion, abduction, external rotation) test leads to groin pain when hip arthritis is present. Joint line tenderness at the knee should also raise suspicion for intrarticular pathology. Radiographs are paramount to diagnosis.

Overuse injuries of the lower extremity are common in athletes performing repetitive knee flexion and extension and can include iliotibial band syndrome. Pain and localized tenderness is typically over the lateral femoral condyle, which is worse with activity and usually relieved with rest. The Ober test starts with the knee flexed and the hip is moved from flexion and abduction to extension and adduction. Imaging is generally negative and can rule out other associated pathology.

DEFICIENCY

Vitamin B12 Deficiency: Neurologic effects of Vitamin B12 deficiency include limb weakness and peripheral neuropathy. Patients often describe paresthesia in their feet and distal lower limbs. Incongruous hematological and neurological effects should raise suspicion of a Vitamin B12 deficiency. Macrocytic anemia is a key finding. A diagnosis can be made based on a serum cobalamin <148 µmol/l in the presence of neurologic symptoms. A serum cobalamin <148 µmol/l with elevated serum homocysteine or methylmalonic acid (MMA) is also indicative of a Vitamin B12 deficiency.[27]

AUTOIMMUNE

HIV/AIDS: Distal symmetric polyneuropathy is one of the most common neurologic findings found in patients with a positive history of Human Immunodeficiency Virus (HIV). The chief complaint is usually sensory loss. Patients may present with a burning neuropathic pain found in a "stocking-glove" distribution. Distal tendon reflexes are often diminished, as are responses to light touch and pinprick. Pain and paresthesia is commonly found in the soles of the feet.[28] Lower limb weakness is less common. Nerve conduction studies show decreased function of sensory and motor nerves in a fashion consistent with Wallerian degradation. Blood tests should be performed to exclude other forms of neuropathy.

Guillain-Barré Syndrome: Patients suffering from Guillain-Barré syndrome typically present with an acute ascending limb weakness.[10] Patients may even progress to respiratory failure as a result of weakness of the diaphragm. Symptoms generally peak around 4 weeks following onset. The cause to this disorder is not entirely known, but approximately two thirds of patients describe a previous infection. Upon physical exam, patients may complain of loss of sensation, paresthesia, and may demonstrate diminished reflexes in self-described weak areas. Severe fatigue is also a common finding. Nerve conduction study results are consistent with peripheral neuropathy. Lumbar puncture to sample CSF is used to rule out infection or cancer, and cytoalbuminic dissociation, increased protein concentration with decreased cell count, may be present.[29] The majority of patients recover motor and sensory function, but a small subset of GBS patients may experience lasting deficits.

ANATOMIC

Spinal Cord/Nerve Compression: Radiculopathy, myelopathy, cauda equina syndrome: Radiculopathy caused by compression of the lumbar nerve roots leads to pain, weakness, and sensory deficits in the lower extremities. L2 radiculopathy leads to symptoms down the medial thigh. An L3 radiculopathy leads to radiating pain into anterior thigh and knee. L2 and L3 roots primarily innervate the hip flexors and adductors, via the femoral and obturator nerves respectively. Hip flexion and adduction tests should therefore be tested clinically. In an L4 radiculopathy there is pain and parasthesias in the medial leg radiating to the medial malleolus. In the case of the L3 and L4 radiculopathies there may be an absent or attenuated patellar reflex. L5 radiculopathy classically involves pain and parasthesias that radiate from the lateral thigh and lower lateral leg into the first dorsal toe web space and there is weakness in great toe extension and dorsiflexion of the ankle. A positive Straight Leg Raise (SLR) test, Lasègue's sign, provokes pain when the patient's leg is raised while supine, suggestive of L5 or S1 compression.[30] In an S1 radiculopathy there is also weakness of the foot with plantar flexion and eversion. The pain and radiating parasthesias classically travel through the posterior thigh, posterior leg, lateral plantar foot, and toes. Reflexes of the Achilles tendon may be absent or attenuated.[13] Radiographs may demonstrate skeletal changes, such as loss of intervertebral space, changes in curvature, and/or degenerative changes. MRIs are both very sensitive and specific for identifying lumbar radiculopathies due to disc herniation and are essential for determining a surgical plan.[30]

Cauda equina injuries may be associated with radicular injuries that affect the leg. Signs and symptoms specific to the sacral nerves include: bowel, bladder, and sexual dysfunction. Cauda equine syndrome is a surgical emergency. The most prominent symptoms occurring are urinary retention or incontinence. The bladder symptoms are noticed sooner than sexual dysfunction or bowel changes. A rectal exam looking for decreased or absent tone and sensation is mandatory.

Neurogenic claudication mimics the symptoms of vascular claudication. The pain in neurogenic claudication is present while standing or ambulating and can be relieved by sitting. Pain from vascular claudication could attenuate with resting while standing. There is often no abnormality with peripheral pulses with neurogenic claudication.

Referred Pain: Pain from viscera may appear along a vague dermatomal distribution due to the convergence of primary cutaneous and visceral afferents on the same secondary neuron within the dorsal horn of the spinal cord.[10] Referred pain is generally described in vague terms and may also present with skin reddening due to inflammation. Pain from the colon and/or appendix generally appears in the lower abdomen, with appendicitis usually localized to the right side T10 dermatome. Kidney pain is referred to the lower back or groin area, from L1 to L2, while bladder and ureter pain is found more along the perineal region, L1. Pain from reproductive organs may be described along the T10-T12 dermatomes (Fig. 6.1).[10,31]

TRAUMA

Fracture: Fractures are almost always a result from an acute traumatic injury. Pain, limited range of motion, refusal to bear weight and deformity of the extremity may be present. Generally there is no sensory abnormality unless a peripheral nerve is damaged. Hip fractures are the most common fracture that leads to hospitalization. The possibility of a hip fracture increases with age, presence of osteoporosis or known systemic malignancy. Stinchfield test reproduces hip joint pain with a resisted straight leg raise.[2] There may be pain with passive log roll of the leg by the examiner. Be wary of chronic groin, buttock, or thigh pain with weight bearing in long distance runners as this may portend a hip stress fracture. Medial tibial stress syndrome, also known as shin splints, occurs in runners, and athletes often involved in jumping sports or long distance running. Frequently there is dysfunction of the tibialis posterior, tibialis anterior, and soleus muscles. The pain is often diffuse along the mid distal tibia, and is worsened with activity. This may advance to a tibial stress fracture if repetitive activity continues without rest.

Compartment Syndrome: A compartment syndrome occurs when the pressures within the leg compartment become so great that it interferes with blood flow. This can threaten the viability of the limb and is a surgical emergency. The six P's can herald a compartment syndrome: pain, parasthesias, pallor,

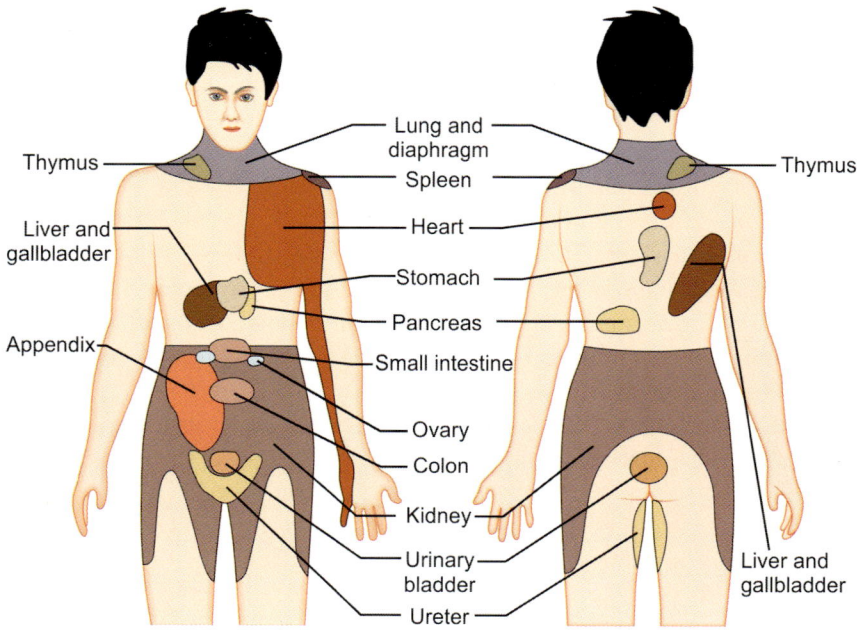

Fig. 6.1: Referred dermatomal patterns of pain from viscera.

partial paralysis, pulselessness, and ploikiothermia. There is swelling of the leg, with severe pain, and tenderness to palpation of the muscular compartment. Also, there may be decreased sensation in the region due to either compromised blood flow or direct compression of peripheral nerves. There is frequently pain upon passive stretching of the muscle. Pulses distal to the compartment may be diminished, but is rarely seen clinically.[13]

Ligament/Tendon Disruption: Stressing the medial and lateral collateral ligaments tests for stability. Palpation of the medial and lateral joint lines helps diagnose synovitis as well as meniscal tears. The anterior drawer test and Lachman test evaluate for ACL (anterior cruciate ligament) disruption. The posterior drawer test evaluates for posterior cruciate ligament stability.[2] A meniscal tear may lead to joint line tenderness. McMurray's Test will lead to clicking and pain during knee extension along with leg rotation for medial or lateral meniscus injuries. The joints themselves may have swelling and effusions present.[2,13]

TOXINS

Alcohol: Polyneuropathy is a common finding among chronic alcohol users and involves a gradual onset of symptoms. Early symptoms of alcoholic-nutritional polyneuropathy include sensory loss in the distal lower limbs and decreased or absent reflexes.[32] As neuropathy progresses, more lower motor neuron signs become evident including atrophy and muscle weakness. Symptoms are generally symmetric and begin distally and include gait imbalance, burning pain, and numbness. Patients are also at increase risk for compression syndromes, including Carpal Tunnel syndrome and compression of the peroneal nerve as it crosses the head of the fibula.[33] A history of alcohol abuse is key in making an accurate diagnosis in such patients.

Medications: Polyneuropathy is a common side effect of many medications. Medically-induced toxic neuropathies vary in their presentation, based on the types of neurons affected, the pattern of symptoms, the dose administered, and nerve conduction study and EMG (Electromyography) information.[34] Common agents include antibiotics, chemotherapeutic drugs, immunosuppressive drugs, and cardiovascular-related treatment.

ENDOCRINE

Diabetic Neuropathy: Diabetic neuropathy is a common complication caused by chronic hyperglycemia. Commonly, it presents as a burning pain in the plantar aspects of the feet. There can be decreased sensation along the affected nerves. Reflexes may be diminished. In the diabetic population there may also be overlapping vascular disease with diminished pulses.[13]

Electrolyte Abnormalities—Hypokalemia, Hypocalcaemia: Clinical signs of hypokalemia include severe, ascending muscle weakness that may lead to flaccid paralysis, cramps, areflexia, and rhabdomyolysis.[35,36] Severity of symptoms depends on serum potassium levels. Patients are generally asymptomatic at 3.0 – 3.5 meq/liter and become progressively more symptomatic as levels fall below 3.0 meq/liter.[36] Blood lab values are indicated to differentiate between other very similar patterns of weakness, including hyperkalemia and Guillain-Barré syndrome. Cardiac arrhythmias may also be present.

While patients may be asymptomatic, acute hypocalcemia often presents with severe symptoms and requires rapid treatment. Neuromuscular excitability is the classic symptom and presents as fasiculations, weakness, spasms, or numbness.[36,37] Neuromuscular excitability may only be visible when provoked. Two useful tests for this are Chvostek's sign, facial muscle spasms upon parotid gland stimulation, and Trosseau's sign, carpopedal spasm with blood pressure cuff inflation.[37] Elevated levels of Parathyroid Hormone (PTH) provide key information in hypocalcemic patients, along with other serologic values.

CONCLUSION

The role of the spine surgeon is to use the clinical picture presented to make an accurate diagnosis, plan the appropriate treatment, and execute the necessary procedure. A patient's leg pain may present through numerous mechanisms, and selecting the correct underlying cause may prove difficult. We have provided here an overview of common causes of leg pain and the clinical clues that may lead to an accurate diagnosis. A complete exam should involve sensory and motor testing, and lab diagnostic tests should be included when indicated. Radiographic, CT, and MRI studies are crucial in making certain diagnoses. In sum, a complete understanding of the anatomy and physiology of the spine, coupled with the material we have presented here, should aid in making an accurate diagnosis for leg pain.

REFERENCES

1.   Miller A, Davis BA, DiCuccio Heckert K. The 3-minute musculoskeletal and peripheral nerve exam. New York, NY: Demos Medical; 2009.

2.   Mengel MB, Schwiebert LP, eds. Family medicine: Ambulatory care and prevention. 4th ed. New York: Lange Medical Books/McGraw-Hill; 2005.

3.   Mallick IH, Thoufeeq MH, Rajendran TP. Iliopsoas abscesses. Postgrad Med J. 2004;80(946):459-462. doi: 10.1136/pgmj.2003.017665.

4.   Turecki MB, Taljanovic MS, Stubbs AY, et al. Imaging of musculoskeletal soft tissue infections. Skeletal Radiol. 2010;39(10):957-971. doi: 10.1007/s00256-009-0780-0.

5.   Hirschmann JV, Raugi GJ. Lower limb cellulitis and its mimics: part I. lower limb cellulitis. J Am Acad Dermatol. 2012;67(2):163.e1-12; quiz 175-6. doi: 10.1016/j.jaad.2012.03.024.

6.   Mathew AJ, Ravindran V. Infections and arthritis. Best Pract Res Clin Rheumatol. 2014;28(6):935-959. doi: 10.1016/j.berh.2015.04.009 [doi].

7.   Lee YH, Bae SC, Song GG. Diagnostic accuracy of anti-MCV and anti-CCP antibodies in rheumatoid arthritis : a meta-analysis. Z Rheumatol. 2015. doi: 10.1007/s00393-015-1598-x.

8.   McCarty DJ, Hollander JL. Identification of urate crystals in gouty synovial fluid. Ann Intern Med. 1961;54:452-460.

9.   Greenspan A. Benign bone-forming lesions: osteoma, osteoid osteoma, and osteoblastoma. Clinical, imaging, pathologic, and differential considerations. Skeletal Radiol. 1993;22(7):485-500.

10.   Nolte J, ed. The human brain : An introduction to its functional anatomy. 6th ed ed. St. Louis: Mosby; 2008.

11.   Tipton JS. Obturator neuropathy. Curr Rev Musculoskelet Med. 2008;1(3-4):234-237. doi: 9030 [pii].

12.   Yuen EC, Olney RK, So YT. Sciatic neuropathy: Clinical and prognostic features in 73 patients. Neurology. 1994;44(9):1669-1674.

13.   Neuhauser TS. The complete history and physical exam guide. Saunders; 2003.

14.   Kopell HP, Thompson WAL. Knee pain due to saphenous-nerve entrapment. N Engl J Med. 1960;263(7):351-353. http://dx.doi.org/10.1056/NEJM19600818 2630707. doi: 10.1056/NEJM196008182630707.

15.   Anselmi SJ. Common peroneal nerve compression. J Am Podiatr Med Assoc. 2006;96(5):413-417. doi: 96/5/413 [pii].

16.   Paraskevas G, Tzika M, Natsis K. Entrapment of the superficial peroneal nerve: an anatomical insight. J Am Podiatr Med Assoc. 2014. doi: 10.7547/12-151.1.

17.   Genc B, Solak A, Kalaycioglu S, Sahin N. Distal tibial osteochondroma causing fibular deformity and deep peroneal nerve entrapment neuropathy: A case report. Acta Orthop Traumatol Turc. 2014;48(4):463-466. doi: 10.3944/AOTT.2014.2741.

18. Bailie DS, Kelikian AS. Tarsal tunnel syndrome: diagnosis, surgical technique, and functional outcome. Foot Ankle Int. 1998;19(2):65-72.

19. Paraskevas GK, Natsis K, Tzika M, Ioannidis O. Fascial entrapment of the sural nerve and its clinical relevance. Anat Cell Biol. 2014;47(2):144-147. doi: 10.5115/acb.2014.47.2.144.

20. Krajewski KM, Lewis RA, Fuerst DR, et al. Neurological dysfunction and axonal degeneration in charcot-marie-tooth disease type 1A. Brain. 2000;123 (Pt 7) (Pt 7):1516-1527.

21. McArthur KS, Quinn TJ, Dawson J, Walters MR. Diagnosis and management of transient ischaemic attack and ischaemic stroke in the acute phase. BMJ. 2011;342:d1938. doi: 10.1136/bmj.d1938.

22. Purrucker JC, Hametner C, Engelbrecht A, Bruckner T, Popp E, Poli S. Comparison of stroke recognition and stroke severity scores for stroke detection in a single cohort. J Neurol Neurosurg Psychiatry. 2014. doi: jnnp-2014-309260 [pii].

23. Balami JS, Chen RL, Buchan AM. Stroke syndromes and clinical management. QJM. 2013;106(7):607-615. doi: 10.1093/qjmed/hct057.

24. McDonald WI, Compston A, Edan G, et al. Recommended diagnostic criteria for multiple sclerosis: guidelines from the international panel on the diagnosis of multiple sclerosis. Ann Neurol. 2001;50(1):121-127.

25. Shayesteh-Azar M, Kariminasab MH, Saravi MS, et al. A survey of severity and distribution of musculoskeletal pain in multiple sclerosis patients; a cross-sectional study. Arch Bone Jt Surg. 2015;3(2):114-118.

26. Rowland LP, Shneider NA. Amyotrophic lateral sclerosis. N Engl J Med. 2001;344(22):1688-1700. doi: 10.1056/NEJM200105313442207.

27. Shipton MJ, Thachil J. Vitamin B12 deficiency—a 21st century perspective. Clin Med. 2015;15(2):145-150. doi: 10.7861/clinmedicine.15-2-145.

28. Cornblath DR, McArthur JC. Predominantly sensory neuropathy in patients with AIDS and AIDS-related complex. Neurology. 1988;38(5):794-796.

29. Yuki N, Hartung HP. Guillain-Barré syndrome. N Engl J Med. 2012;366(24):2294-2304. doi: 10.1056/NEJMra1114525.

30. Suri P, Rainville J, Katz JN, et al. The accuracy of the physical examination for the diagnosis of midlumbar and low lumbar nerve root impingement. Spine (Phila Pa 1976). 2011;36(1):63-73. doi: 10.1097/BRS.0b013e3181c953cc.

31. Autonomic reflexes and homeostasis. http://cnx.org/contents/0bae7483-e6a1-47eb-8571-723ea8ed4131@2/Autonomic-Reflexes-and-Homeost. Updated 2013. Accessed 04/03, 2015.

32. Hawley RJ, Kurtzke JF, Armbrustmacher VW, Saini N, Manz H. The course of alcoholic-nutritional peripheral neuropathy. Acta Neurol Scand. 1982;66(5):582-589.

33. Kemppainen R, Juntunen J, Hillbom M. Drinking habits and peripheral alcoholic neuropathy. Acta Neurol Scand. 1982;65(1):11-18.

34. Morrison B, Chaudhry V. Medication, toxic, and vitamin-related neuropathies. Continuum (Minneap Minn). 2012;18(1):139-160. doi: 10.1212/01.CON.0000411565.49332.84.

35. Comi G, Testa D, Cornelio F, Comola M, Canal N. Potassium depletion myopathy: a clinical and morphological study of six cases. Muscle Nerve. 1985;8(1):17-21. doi: 10.1002/mus.880080104.

36. Knochel JP. Neuromuscular manifestations of electrolyte disorders. Am J Med. 1982;72(3):521-535.

37. Cooper MS, Gittoes NJ. Diagnosis and management of hypocalcaemia. BMJ. 2008;336(7656):1298-1302. doi: 10.1136/bmj.39582.589433.BE.

CHAPTER 7

Bowel/Bladder Incontinence, Retention, and Saddle Anesthesia

Heidi M Hullinger, Rex AW Marco

CHIEF COMPLAINT/HISTORY

Patients presenting with bowel and/or bladder dysfunction must be carefully evaluated to determine if spinal pathology could be the cause. Patients may complain of a constellation of bowel and bladder symptomatology, or their complaints may be isolated to either urinary or bowel dysfunction alone. They can present with a sudden, acute onset of symptoms or with a more insidious onset.

Urinary dysfunction ranges from frank retention to complete urinary incontinence. Patients with retention may note severe suprapubic pain or alternatively painless suprapubic distention along with unsuccessful attempts to urinate. Frequently, when the bladder becomes overextended, a patient will experience overflow incontinence, with small amounts of urine being spilled when the bladder can no longer accommodate the large volume. On the other end of the spectrum is complete urinary incontinence; patients may only recognize that they have voided when they feel that they have soiled themselves. This may be constant, or they may be able to intermittently sense their urine and control it. Patients may also note milder forms of urinary dysfunction, ranging from increasing strain when initiating a urinary stream to difficulty with cutting off a urinary stream.

Bowel dysfunction tends to present with incontinence as opposed to retention/constipation. Patients may be aware of stool when it is higher within the rectal vault but then not be able to sense when it travels more distally; they also may note that it is more difficult for them to bear down to control the anal sphincter. If the symptoms are of more chronic onset, patients may be able to manage their bowel movements by using the restroom once they feel stool within the vault. However, when the symptoms are of acute onset, patients often have frank bowel incontinence.

Patients generally notice saddle anesthesia when they wipe themselves following using the restroom; they may note either complete numbness with inability to feel the toilet paper, or they may note a hypersensitivity or other altered sensation. It also can manifest by an inability to sense a bowel or bladder accident until they have voided a large volume.

Some patients utilize external stimuli to aid with bowel and bladder dysfunction, particularly when it is mild or of insidious onset. In the case of urinary retention, they sometimes find relief via manual pressure on the bladder, forcing out the urinary stream. Patients may utilize digital manipulation of the rectum; this is most common in those who have had a gradual onset of bowel incontinence. These patients can utilize this technique to void once they feel stool higher in the rectal vault to avoid losing a bowel movement by accident.

DIFFERENTIAL DIAGNOSES

It is important to distinguish neurogenic urinary and bowel symptomatology from more common conditions such as urge or stress incontinence in females, overflow incontinence due to prostate hypertrophy in males, or gastrointestinal conditions such as inflammatory bowel syndrome, irritable bowel disease, or viral illness. Patients with urge incontinence will note that they are aware when they need to void their urine, but that it can be difficult to make it to the bathroom on time. Meanwhile, stress incontinence, which is due to weakness of the pelvic floor, involves the loss of a small amount of urine when intra-abdominal pressure is raised, such as during a sneeze or a cough. Primary gastrointestinal (GI) conditions can be accompanied by either blood in the stool or a softening of normal stool consistency; in addition, patients will feel the urge to defecate but may occasionally have difficulty making it to the restroom in time.

If the above conditions can be reasonably ruled out, the focus can be turned toward possible neurologic causes. It is important to recognize that the effect that spinal pathology has on bowel and bladder function can be somewhat variable, in part due to the complex interplay of autonomic and voluntary control of the bowel and bladder. The signal for voluntary control of urinary function travels through the spinal cord and then via the pudendal nerve, with contributions from S2-S4, to the external sphincter; this is responsible for retaining urine despite an urge to urinate. Activation of the parasympathetic system also occurs via the S2-S4 roots but is instead responsible for promoting voiding. Meanwhile, the sympathetic chain, which exits in the T11-L3 segments, promotes urinary retention (Fig. 7.1). In general, therefore, upper motor lesions will lead to urinary incontinence due to a combination of bladder detrusor hyperreflexia and loss of voluntary sphincter control, while lower motor neuron lesions below the conus will lead to retention due to loss of detrusor function as well as unopposed internal sphincter tone.[1] However, it is important to note that due to the interactions of afferent and efferent signals at various levels of the cord and spinal nerves, variations from these "typical presentations" are not uncommon. In

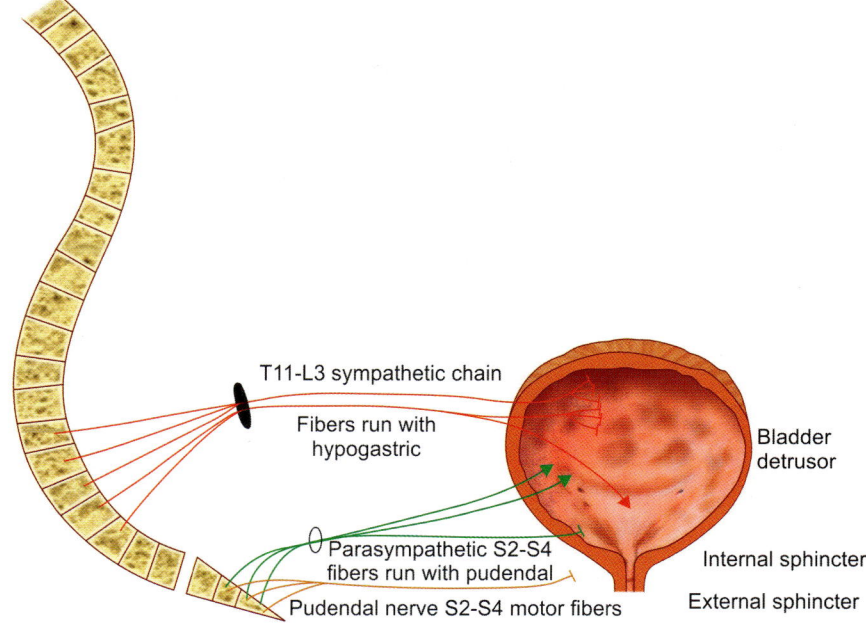

Fig. 7.1: Urinary control involves neurologic signals to the bladder detrusor, internal sphincter, and external sphincter. Sympathetic fibers (red) from the thoracolumbar segments run with the hypogastric nerve to promote urinary retention. Parasympathetic fibers (green) from the sacral segments run along the pudendal nerve to promote bladder emptying. Voluntary control of bladder emptying is via motor fibers (yellow) from the sacral segments running within the pudendal nerve.

particular, patients with upper motor neuron dysfunction may have increased external sphincter tone in addition to bladder detrusor hyperactivity and thus manifest with retention; this is discussed in further detail in the section on urodynamic testing.[2]

When patients have a sudden onset of symptoms, the differential includes such acute conditions as cauda equina/conus medullaris syndrome or a fracture causing neurologic compression. Patients with cauda equina syndrome may or may not report an acute traumatic event; the earliest presenting symptom is often urinary retention, which occurs due to loss of the normal neurologic signal to the bladder detrusor muscle. These patients will generally have significant acute back pain, though if they present more than a day after onset, the pain may have partly subsided. In some cases, the patient may also experience bowel incontinence due to loss of voluntary sphincter control; this is a poor prognostic factor. Conus medullaris syndrome can present similarly, though patients may instead experience incontinence due to detrusor hyperactivity.[3] Meanwhile, a frank traumatic injury may also lead to acute bowel or bladder dysfunction. A combination of urinary incontinence and bowel incontinence suggests an upper motor neuron

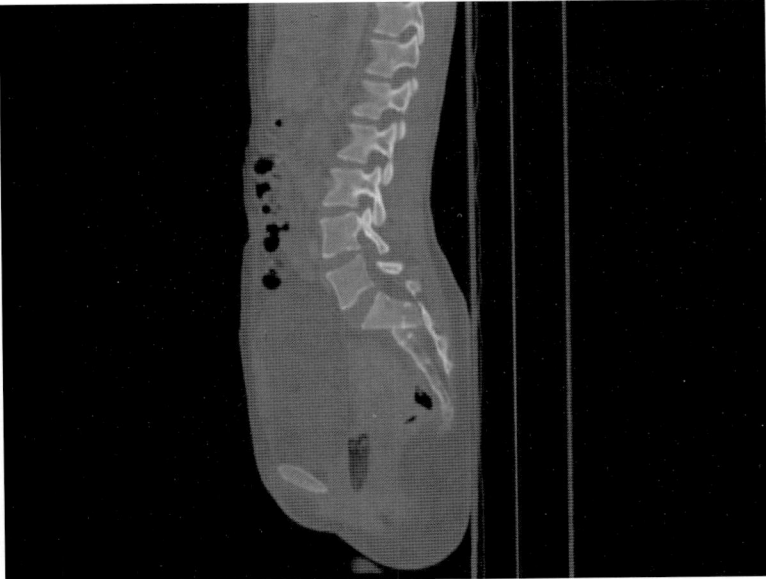

Fig. 7.2: Transverse fracture through S2 with kyphotic deformity; this is associated with high risk of neurologic sequelae including bowel/bladder dysfunction.

lesion such as a cervical or thoracic injury, while, as noted above, urinary retention is usually a sign of lower motor neuron pathology. Zone 2 and zone 3 sacral injuries, particularly when displaced, can present with retention. Transverse sacral fractures present an even higher risk of bowel and bladder dysfunction, particularly when there is kyphotic deformity that can develop at the site of injury (Fig. 7.2). Bowel and bladder dysfunction in this setting has a particularly poor prognosis.[4]

Patients with constitutional symptoms such as weight loss or loss of appetite or who have onset of severe axial pain may have a tumor causing cord compression or, less frequently, a sacral tumor causing sacral nerve dysfunction. Tumors may be metastatic or primary, with the most common primary tumors with metastases to the bone arising from the prostate, breast, lung, kidney, and hematopoietic system. In the sacrum, the most common primary tumors include chordomas and giant cell tumors (Fig. 7.3).[5] Intradural tumors, whether intra- or extramedullary, may also present with bladder/ bowel dysfunction; the differential includes ependymomas, gliomas, and nerve sheath tumors.

Other intrinsic lesions or pathologies of the spinal cord itself that may lead to bowel/bladder dysfunction via upper motor neuron abnormalities include a tethered cord or a syrinx. While a syrinx may be due to an abnormality such as a tethered cord or Chiari malformation, it may also be idiopathic in etiology.

Nonspinal neurologic diseases may also manifest with autonomic dys-function; demyelinating diseases such as multiple sclerosis or transverse

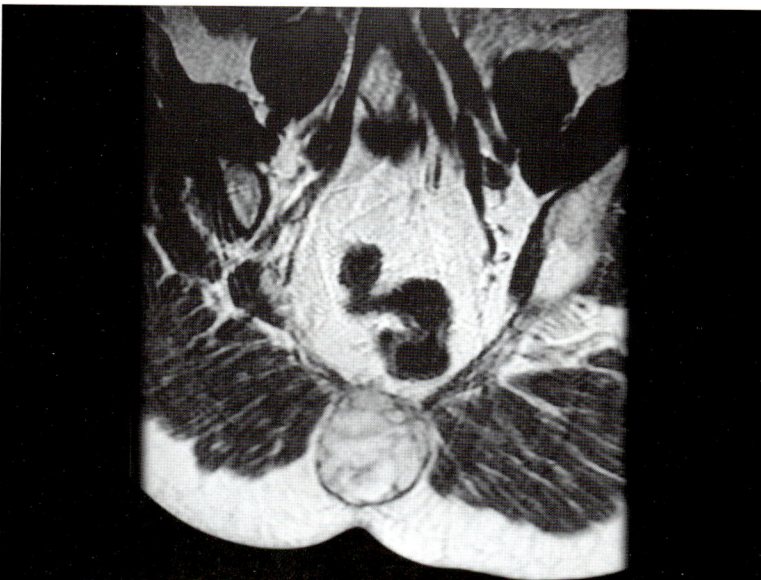

Fig. 7.3: T2-weighted axial image showing a chordoma at the tip of the sacrum, as seen toward the bottom of the image. It has a typically well-circumscribed appearance due to its slow growing nature. While it displays low intensity on T1 images, it is generally of moderate intensity and with some heterogeneity on T2 images, as seen here.

myelitis are high in the differential within this category.[6] Both of these disorders also present with variable lower extremity dysfunction, and therefore can present much like pathology of the spinal column; as will be discussed below, imaging is crucial to differentiate between these entities. Other pathologies such as cerebrovascular insults and Parkinson's disease can have associated urinary dysfunction, generally presenting with a lack of control of the external sphincter leading to incontinence.

EVALUATION

A detailed history with specific questions regarding a patient's bowel/bladder dysfunction can help a practitioner localize the likely source of pathology. As noted above, when bladder dysfunction is combined with bowel dysfunction, a neurologic cause is high on the differential. When the patient also notes altered sensation primarily in the perineum, this points towards a lesion of the cauda equina or the sacrum. When acute, this requires prompt imaging to evaluate for cauda equina syndrome, which will be discussed further below.

There is a broader differential when a patient presents with bladder dysfunction alone. When a patient notes incontinence, it must be delineated whether it is a small amount of urine escaping or whether they have a normal flow but cannot hold it in. The former is due to either pelvic floor weakness or overflow incontinence secondary to urinary retention; patients should be questioned as to whether they can tell if their bladder is full, either by a sense of distention or by noting suprapubic fullness. This is an indicator of overflow incontinence, which can either be due to a structural obstruction such as an enlarged prostate or to dysfunction of the sacral nerve roots with resultant detrusor flaccidity. Patients who are unable to sense distention of the bladder are more likely to have a neurologic basis for their dysfunction.

Meanwhile, patients experiencing a complete inability to hold in their urine are more likely to have upper motor neuron dysfunction, which may be due to pathology within the spinal column or may be due to other neurologic dysfunction such as a cerebrovascular incident or neurologic disease. Patients who are aware that they have to void but have urgency are less likely to have a neurologic origin of dysfunction, though this can be an early symptom of cervical myelopathy. Later in the course of disease, cervical myelopathy can progress to frank urinary incontinence due to upper motor neuron dysfunction and lack of voluntary control over the external sphincter.

A full neurologic exam of the upper and lower extremities should then be performed to further delineate the likely source of dysfunction. If sensory deficits are seen both within the perineum as well as in distributions in the lower extremities, cauda equina syndrome should be high on the differential; motor deficits in the lower extremities can also be seen. While cauda equina and conus medullaris syndrome can present similarly, conus medullaris syndrome is more likely to cause asymmetric lower extremity deficits than cauda equina syndrome. Sensory deficits limited to the perineum, i.e. isolated saddle anesthesia, can be either due to a cauda equina lesion or a sacral lesion such as a tumor. If there is concern for a sacral tumor, direct palpation of the sacrum may in some cases elicit tenderness or even reveal a prominence along the dorsal aspect of the sacrum, particularly in the case of a slow growing tumor such as a chordoma. If there are upper extremity findings or pathologic reflexes such as a Hoffman's sign or upgoing Babinski reflex, the pathology is more likely located within the spinal cord or the cerebral cortex, so attention should be turned to these regions.

Palpation of the bladder can help confirm whether a patient's low-volume loss of urine is due to urinary retention leading to overflow incontinence. Suprapubic fullness, whether painful to palpation or not, indicates an inability to properly void, which can be due to lack of proper detrusor contractility and/or to continuous internal sphincter contraction. This pattern is most frequently seen in pathologies within the cauda equina due to imbalance of the autonomic nervous system, as sympathetic signals promote retention and overwhelm the ineffectual signals of the parasympathetic nervous system.

A rectal exam is of utmost importance, and it includes several components: testing sensation to light touch in the perianal region, assessing for the anal wink and bulbocavernosus reflexes, and determining both resting rectal tone and ability to bear down. Decreased perianal sensation is a component of saddle anesthesia; sensation in the rest of the perineum as well as lower extremities should subsequently be evaluated if not already done. The anal wink reflex is evaluated by applying light pressure at the base of the anus as one is preparing to do a digital rectal exam; if the anal wink is intact, there will be an involuntary contraction of the external sphincter. Meanwhile, the bulbocavernosus reflex is assessed while performing a digital rectal exam by pulling on a Foley catheter to gently apply traction to the bladder neck; contraction of the internal sphincter indicates an intact bulbocavernosus reflex. The above reflexes both rely on afferent sensory feedback as well as efferent output; abnormalities are typically due either to an interruption in function of the lower sacral nerve roots or to spinal shock in a patient in the early stage of acute spinal cord injury. Resting rectal tone is a function of the sympathetic nerve roots; a decrease in the normal tone thus implies dysfunction of these fibers, which occurs in injuries occurring at or above the thoracolumbar junction. Ability to bear down, meanwhile, is governed by a voluntary signal traveling down the spinal cord to the external sphincter via the pudendal nerve. It can thus be disrupted by interruption of the signal either within the cord or within the sacral nerve roots that provide fibers to the pudendal nerve, namely S2-S4.

IMAGING

Based on the history and examination, if there is any suspicion for a neurologic origin of bowel/bladder dysfunction, appropriate spinal imaging should be performed. If the symptoms are of acute onset, this imaging must be performed in an urgent fashion. In the case of suspicion for cauda equina/conus medullaris syndrome, a magnetic resonance imaging (MRI) should be performed of the lumbar spine immediately; if the patient cannot undergo a MRI, a computed tomography (CT) myelogram is a reasonable alternative. This imaging should extend all the way up to the thoracolumbar junction to ensure that pathology at the level of the conus is not missed. A MRI will show whether there are any compressive lesions such as a large central disk herniation (Figs. 7.4A and B), a tumor with significant canal involvement, or an epidural hematoma. There is a small subset of patients who can have cauda equina syndrome without having any evidence of a compressive lesion on imaging, namely patients who have recently undergone a lumbar microdiskectomy. While post-diskectomy cauda equina syndrome is a well-recognized entity, the etiology is still not well understood; it is postulated to be due to post-operative tissue edema.[7] Thus, while a post-diskectomy patient with new onset of bowel/bladder dysfunction should always have imaging to rule out a repeat extrusion, a lack of compressive pathology on imaging does not necessarily rule out cauda equina syndrome in these patients.

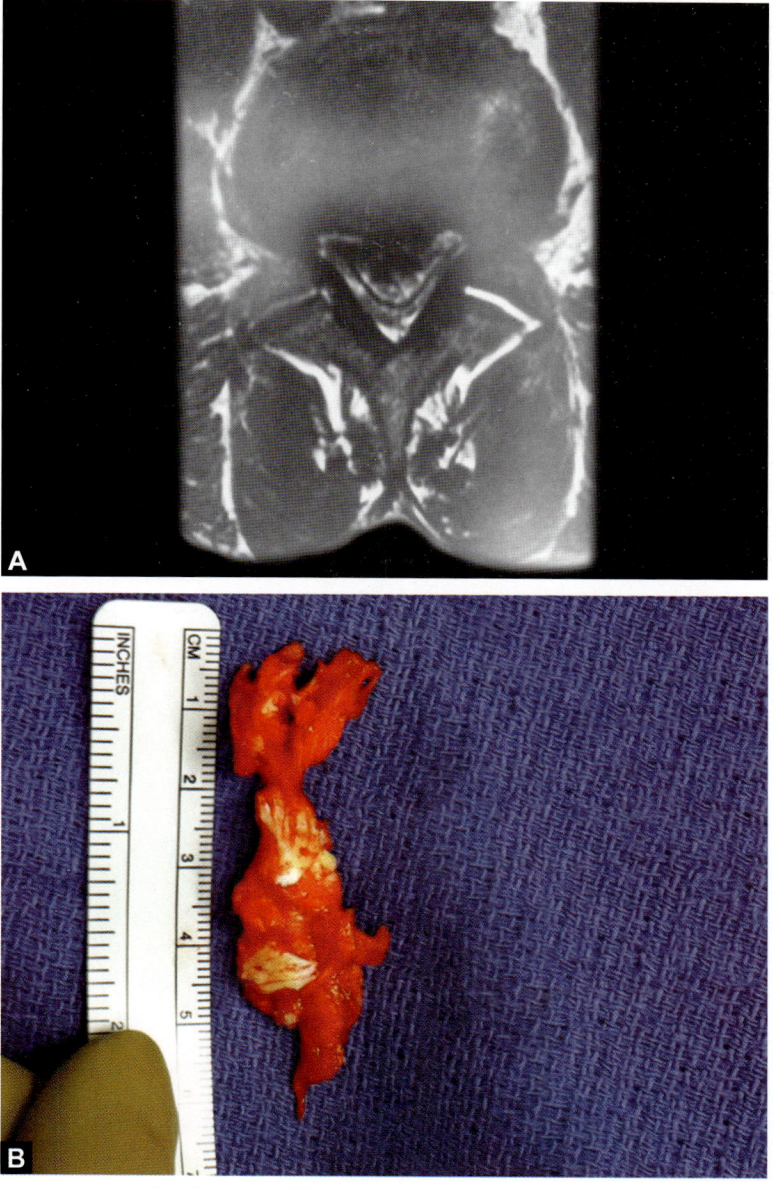

Figs. 7.4A and B: (A) On these T2-weighted images, a large central disk herniation has compressed the cauda equina to such an extent that CSF signal is nearly absent. (B) The large disk fragment from 4A removed during urgent decompression.

Patients with acute trauma are generally best initially evaluated with a CT scan as opposed to MRI, since bony injuries are best evaluated on CT imaging. While fractures can be well identified on CT imaging, more subtle findings such as an increase in interspinous distance or facet diastasis, subluxation, or incongruity should alert a practitioner that there may be

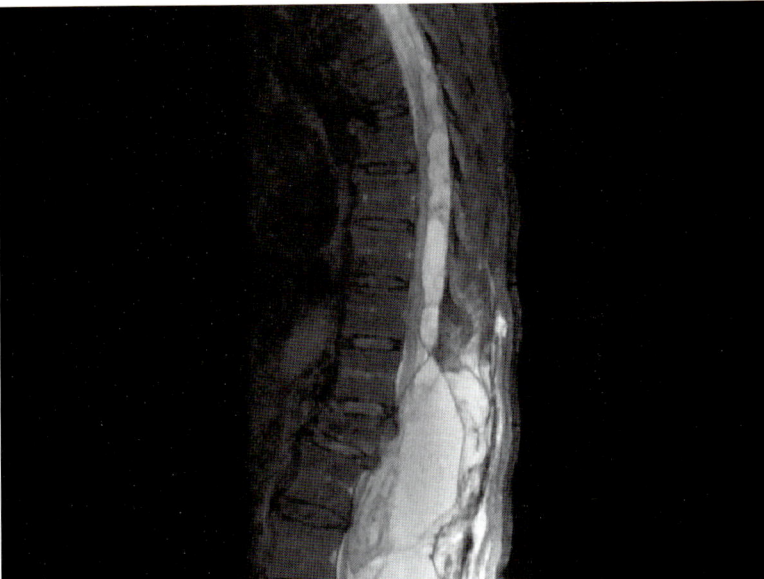

Fig. 7.5: These sagittal T2-weighted images show an acute epidural hematoma that has accumulated after a recent decompression. It can be seen as a loculated hyperintense collection separate from the CSF that extends up to the mid-thoracic region.

significant soft tissue disruption that has led to spinal injury. MRI can be useful to further delineate extent of soft tissue injury, evaluate for an epidural hematoma, or look for cord edema indicative of significant cord injury. In the case of an incomplete spinal cord injury, hemorrhage within the spinal cord, as represented by hypointensity on T2, portends worse prognosis for recovery of neural function than the hyperintensity of edema within the cord.

Patients without a known trauma but who present with sudden onset of neurologic decline including bowel/bladder dysfunction raise concern for either a cord lesion or an intracranial abnormality. X-rays may be obtained initially to look for an obvious bony lesion, but regardless, a MRI should be performed on an urgent basis and should not be delayed in the name of obtaining a screening X-ray. Possible etiologies include an epidural hematoma, a tumor causing cord compression, or a severe central cord syndrome from a low energy injury in a patient with underlying cervical stenosis. An acute epidural hematoma will be hyperintense on T2 and will be seen as a separate collection within the cerebrospinal fluid (CSF) (Fig. 7.5), while a subacute hematoma will be iso- or hypointense on T2. Of note, epidural hematomas may be seen after an invasive procedure or may occur spontaneously in patients on anticoagulation or with a bleeding diathesis. Tumors in the spinal column are most often seen originating within the vertebral body; as the lesion expands, it can press into the spinal canal and cause cord compression. Most commonly, the posterior longitudinal

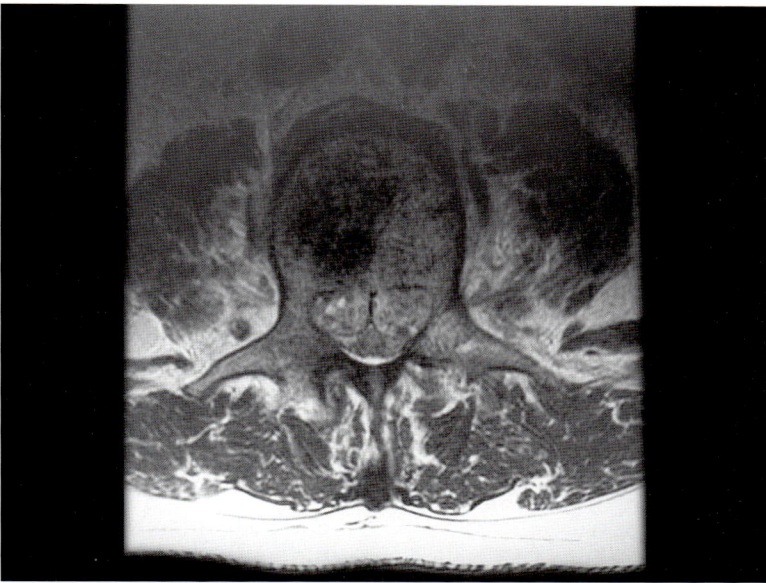

Fig. 7.6: This T2-weighted axial image demonstrates the "buttocks sign" seen when an expansile mass, most typically a metastatic lesion, presses against the PLL and stenoses the spinal canal. In this case, a metastatic lesion has compressed the cauda equina to the point that CSF signal is no longer visible amongst individual nerve roots.

ligament (PLL) will remain intact but will deform as the tumor encroaches upon the spinal canal, creating the pathognomonic "buttocks sign" (Fig. 7.6). Imaging in central cord syndrome will show severe cervical canal stenosis and accompanying cord edema in the region of injury; soft tissue injuries such as ligamentous disruption can also be seen.

In patients with more insidious onset of bowel/bladder dysfunction without an obvious causative factor, X-rays should be obtained in the office as an initial screening study. These can be examined for facet arthropathy and disk collapse that are seen in lumbar or cervical stenosis, as well as for any bony lesions concerning for a spinal tumor. An MRI can then be performed on an outpatient basis to further assess the extent of any visualized stenosis, to evaluate a bony lesion, or to look for another etiology, assuming there is not severe enough neurologic involvement to warrant admission to the hospital for an inpatient workup. In the absence of stenosis or a bony lesion, the MRI should be scrutinized for intrinsic cord abnormalities such as a syrinx, which can occur in isolation or may accompany cord abnormalities such as a tethered cord or an intramedullary spinal cord tumor. MRI findings consistent with a tethered cord include a thickened filum with diameter >2mm and a low-lying conus, particularly if it extends to or below L2. Findings such as a spinal lipoma, diastematomyelia (duplicated spinal cord), and myelomeningocele or spina bifida occulta may be seen in conjunction with a tethered cord as well.[8]

Other imaging modalities that may occasionally be useful are positron emission tomography-computed tomography (PET-CT) for additional tumor evaluation, ultrasound, or a contrast imaging study. While ultrasound does not play a role in evaluation of the spine, it can be used to evaluate for bladder distention and thus confirm urinary retention. Meanwhile, an MRI with contrast can be useful in a variety of situations, including further workup of infections and tumors. If there is suspicion for infection such as osteodiskitis and/or an epidural abscess, an MRI with contrast can help confirm this, as there will be contrast uptake in the affected regions; the contrast uptake can also delineate the extent of disease. Contrast also has increased uptake in neoplastic tissue and thus is able to delineate the border of a tumor from surrounding soft tissue. Finally, an MRI with contrast can be considered in the post-diskectomy patient that is presenting with cauda equina symptoms as well, as post-surgical changes will enhance with contrast while a repeat herniation will not. However, if contrast cannot be administered or would delay care, a standard MRI will suffice, as any compressive lesion that is severe enough to cause a cauda equina syndrome should be evident.

FURTHER WORKUP

Lab tests are primarily useful to distinguish between a tumor and infection when a contrast-enhancing, space occupying lesion is seen on imaging studies. Workup of an unknown lesion suspicious for a tumor should include labwork as part of the initial staging to determine a possible source of metastatic disease. Relevant labs include complete blood count (CBC) with differential, prostate-specific antigen (PSA), thyroid stimulating hormone (TSH), urinalysis (UA), alkaline phosphatase as part of complete metabolic panel (CMP), and serum/urine protein electrophoresis (SPEP/UPEP). Erythrocyte sedimentation rate (ESR) and C-reactive protein (CRP) should be sent to assess whether the lesion is an infectious process, though these lab values may also be elevated in certain tumors such as Ewings sarcoma.

Electromyography (EMG) can have utility in the evaluation of a patient with more insidious onset of symptoms, but has no role in more acute onset of dysfunction. An EMG of the lower extremities can detect patterns of neurologic involvement that provide additional information as to the likely anatomic location of the neural dysfunction. It may be particularly useful in cases in which the pattern of bowel/bladder dysfunction does not dovetail with the rest of the neurologic exam, ie if a patient with upper motor neuron signs has urinary retention.

Of particular utility in evaluation of patients with mild or chronic urinary dysfunction is urodynamic testing,[9,10] which can delineate the anatomic abnormalities leading to either retention or incontinence. Typical parameters measured in urodynamic testing include voiding volume (VV), post-void residual (PVR), maximum cystometric capacity (MCC), maximum detrusor pressure, bladder compliance, and maximum flow rate. An increased PVR is indicative of urinary retention, which as discussed earlier, can be due to either increased sphincter tone and/or detrusor flaccidity. If urinary retention is chronic, increased bladder capacity, as represented by the MCC, may be seen. A decrease in detrusor pressure, bladder compliance, and maximum flow rate are all indicative of decreased detrusor function. If findings consistent with urinary retention, ie increased PVR and MCC, are seen in conjunction with an increase in bladder detrusor metrics, the patient likely has detrusor-sphincter dyssynergia (DSD). In these patients, despite detrusor hyperactivity, increased external sphincter tone results in urinary retention. DSD is most commonly seen in patients with spinal cord injury, who have an interruption of the nerve fibers controlling micturition that travel from the pons to the sacral nerve roots; it is unclear why it only manifests in a proportion of spinal cord injury (SCI) patients. Because of the high pressures exerted within the lower urinary tract, there is a high incidence of injury to the urinary tract, including vesico-ureteral reflux and hydronephrosis. Therefore, if DSD is suspected in an SCI patient, urodynamic studies should be performed as confirmation.

CONCLUSION

While effects of spinal pathology on bowel and bladder function can be highly variable, there are specific patterns of dysfunction that can help guide the workup. While upper motor neuron pathologies tend to result in urinary and bowel incontinence, lower motor neuron pathologies often manifest with retention along with perineal anesthesia. A physical exam including a five-point rectal exam (sensation to light touch, anal wink reflex, bulbocavernosus reflex, resting rectal tone and ability to bear down) can further lead the practitioner to focus on either the spinal cord or the spinal nerves at/below conus level. Imaging of the relevant spinal regions can then identify the causative pathology; it should be undertaken urgently when dysfunction is acute, particularly when cauda equina syndrome is suspected. Adjuncts such as EMG or urodynamic studies are most useful in patients with mild or chronic dysfunction, particularly when there are not additional neurologic findings. Finally, it is important to note that while in some patients there can be recovery of more normal function once spinal pathology is addressed, in patients with pathologies such as cauda equina syndrome (CES) with bowel involvement, transverse sacral fractures, or severe spinal cord injury, regaining bowel/bladder function is much less predictable.

REFERENCES

1. Smith MD, Seth JH, Fowler CJ, Miller RF, Panicker JN. Urinary retention for the neurologist. Practical Neurology. Oct 2013;13(5):288-291.
2. Wyndaele JJ, Kovindha A, Madersbacher H, et al. Neurologic urinary incontinence. Neurourology and Urodynamics. 2010;29(1):159-164.

3. Kim SY, Kwon HC, Hyun JK. Detrusor overactivity in patients with cauda equina syndrome. Spine. 2014;39(16):E955-61.

4. Dussa CU, Soni BM. Influence of type of management of transverse sacral fractures on neurological outcome. A case series and review of literature. Spinal Cord. Sep 2008;46(9):590-594.

5. Puri A, Agarwal MG, Shah M, et al. Decision making in primary sacral tumors. The Spine Journal: Official Journal of the North American Spine Society. May 2009;9(5):396-403.

6. Fowler CJ, Dalton C, Panicker JN. Review of neurologic diseases for the urologist. The Urologic Clinics of North America. Nov 2010;37(4):517-526.

7. Spector L, Madigan L, Rhyne A, et al. Cauda Equina Syndrome. J Am Acad Orthop Surg. Aug 2008;16(8):471-9.

8. Raghavan N, Barkovich A, Edwards M, et al. MRI Imaging in the tethered spinal cord syndrome. Am J Roentgenol. Jan/Feb 1989;10:27-36.

9. Cong ML, Gong WM, Zhang QG, et al. Urodynamic study of bladder function for patients with lumbar spinal stenosis treated by surgical decompression. Journal of International Medical Research. 2010;38(3):1149-1155.

10. Lew SM, Kothbauer KF. Tethered cord syndrome: an updated review. Pediatric Neurosurgery. 2007;43(3):236-248.

CHAPTER 8

Neck Pain in Adults

Brian P Calio, Anuj Shah, Troy Mounts

INTRODUCTION

Neck pain is a common complaint tending to occur with increasing frequency after the age of 30 years. Sixty-six percent of adults will experience neck pain during their lifetime with 54% having experienced it during the past 6 months. Luckily, most episodes are short-lived and responsive to non-operative management; however, at any given moment up to 5% of adults are highly disabled by it. Neck pain tends to be more prevalent in patients with a higher education, history of prior injury, a history of headaches, and/or a history of low-back pain.

There is a spectrum of possible causes of neck pain ranging from trauma, muscle strain, visceral referral, and degenerative disk disease in the setting of cervical spondylosis, cervical radiculopathy and myelopathy or a mixture of all of the above. With regards to cervical degenerative disk disease there are three general cervical pain syndromes: (1) cervical radiculopathy, (2) cervical myelopathy, and (3) axial neck pain. Mechanically the neck is designed to give mobility to the head while absorbing multidirectional loads imparted by the weight of the head. Repetitive mechanical strain together with a multitude of external factors and the natural aging process affect the natural progression of disk degeneration. As the water content of the disk decreases and their natural shock absorbing ability is diminished, patients may experience pain in the neck, base of the skull and/or the upper trapezius region. The collapse in disk height that accompanies degeneration places undo stress on the zygapophyseal joints with associated facet capsules, ligaments, musculature, and neural elements. These changes can be acute, as in the setting of trauma, chronic, or acute on chronic accelerating the otherwise natural progression of aging.

HISTORY

When patients present with neck pain, a detailed history and physical exam should be performed to elicit characteristics of the pain in order to narrow the potential sources of pain. Often times the patient perceives the pain as existing primarily within the axial portion of the spine whether it is limited to a focal area or involving a more global region. History of the present condition should focus on the time course and progression of the neck pain, as well as location and severity. The astute physician remains abreast of the patient's comorbid medical issues while being ever wary of red-flag symptoms that could indicate a more serious underlying condition requiring immediate intervention.

Initial treatment of neck pain is generally a multimodal approach with nonsteroidal anti-inflammatory drugs (NSAIDs) and physical therapy. Most patients with axial neck pain without neurologic involvement can be managed entirely nonoperatively. Surgery may be required in cases of vertebral fractures, spinal cord compression and neurologic injury or in the setting of radiculopathy or myelopathy. History and physical exam findings correlated with appropriately ordered and performed diagnostic imaging studies can aid in diagnosis. In general a magnetic resonance imaging (MRI) with age-appropriate degenerative changes in the setting of isolated axial neck pain (without referred pain to arms or other areas of the body) is treated nonoperatively often with successful results.

DIFFERENTIAL DIAGNOSIS

Whiplash

Whiplash is a common type of soft-tissue injury to the cervical spine and supporting structures and is referred to medically as a neck strain or sprain in the absence of instability or neurologic injury. Neck sprain or strain can exist on a spectrum and as a component of a much more severe destabilizing injury. In the US, neck injuries are frequent claims reported to insurance companies representing ~25% of all injury-related claim dollars paid annually.

Many people associate whiplash primarily with motor vehicle accidents (MVAs), but less often whiplash can occur in falls, sports injuries, and other physical collisions. In a car accident, those who are hit from behind ("rear-ended") are most at risk for whiplash. In a whiplash accident, the cervical spine is forced into an "S-shaped" curve rather than the normal lordotic "C-shape". The lower cervical spine is bent back and the upper spine is bent forward causing the potential for injury to the ligaments, disks, and joints in that area. The most common cause of chronic neck pain post-whiplash is believed to be injury to the zygapophyseal joints.

Damage to soft tissues supporting the neck presents as diffuse neck pain, and can include shoulder and back pain as well. These symptoms may present immediately or be delayed a few days post-event. Headaches at the base of the skull and dizziness are also common. It is important to understand the mechanism of injury, where the impact came from, if seatbelts were worn, if airbags deployed, and if loss of consciousness occurred. Soon after the incident, patients may show limited range of motion in all planes.

Based on the history and physical, additional imaging may be necessary to clear the cervical spine to rule out fractures and other nerve and spinal cord injuries. Plain radiographs are commonly used for patients as a first imaging option. In the setting of concomitant injuries it is important to consider the effect of a distracting injury when evaluating the cervical spine. Large areas of soft-tissue injury, long bone fractures, pelvis fractures, etc. can distract the patient from a severe destabilizing injury of their cervical spine. In the setting of a distracting injury, an appropriate workup according to the Advanced Trauma Life Support (ATLS) and hospital guidelines should ensue. This workup radiographically includes anterior-posterior (AP)/lateral radiographs of the cervical spine, and often computed tomography (CT) scanning.

A patient presenting following a trauma with isolated neck pain in the absence of any distracting injuries should be evaluated with AP and lateral radiographs of the cervical spine, and/or CT scan. Flexion and extension views of the cervical spine are not performed at the time of initial evaluation after trauma, as unappreciated instability may be missed in the setting of paraspinal cervical spasm. Radiographs can uncover cervical spine injury or abnormalities, but it should be noted that they are non-diagnostic in many cases. In the setting of normal AP and lateral cervical spine radiographs and CT with continued neck pain, the patient should remain in a rigid cervical collar and seen as an outpatient for flexion and extension views of the cervical spine. Neck pain and consequent muscle spasm can limit the telling motion of a destabilizing injury and result in a false negative study. In the setting of suspected nerve root or spinal cord injury or cervical spine fracture, a CT and MRI help to elucidate the pathology and direct management.

Recently there has been a shift towards increasing motion after traumatic events to expedite the healing process. Physical therapy may include range of motion exercises as a primary focus. Treatment may also include pain medications, NSAIDs, muscle relaxants, and antidepressants, whereas previous treatment included a soft collar to immobilize the neck.

For most patients with neck strains and sprains, the prognosis is good. The pain typically resolves within a few days or weeks. After 12 months, 1 in 5 patients remain symptomatic with 5% of patients complaining of severe pain.

Cervical Degenerative Disk Disease

Cervical disk degeneration disease (DDD) is a common cause of neck pain and can predispose patients to acute cervical disk injuries. Patients present primarily with a stiff neck and may also complain of shooting/stabbing or burning pain, numbness, tingling, or even upper extremity weakness due to irritation and/or pinching of one or more cervical nerve root(s). Symptoms in most patients are short-lived, but in some cases can result in chronic pain. Over the course of a 10-year period, studies have shown that 79% of patients have a decrease in pain, while 43% are completely free of pain; however, 32% have moderate or severe residual pain. Typically chronic symptoms are directly related to the amount of physical activity (e.g. use of shoulders, arms, and neck) performed.

Degenerative disk changes may simply reflect a mechanism of normal aging and do not necessarily indicate disease. While attributable to age-related changes in many cases, DDD can also be affected by physical activity, poor nutrition, smoking, and even genetics. Typically disks begin the degeneration process in the 2nd decade of life. A common consequence of degeneration is radial tearing of the annulus, beginning with the interior of the annulus and extending to the outer, pain-sensitive areas of the annulus. Studies have shown that significant annular tears can escape MRI detection.

Cervical DDD may present with chronic intermittent neck pain, exacerbated by certain activities and positions and may be accompanied by upper extremity pain. It is important, though sometimes difficult, to distinguish referred pain from radicular pain or pain due to nerve irritation and/or compression. During the physical exam, patients may be asked to perform cervical flexion, and lateral bending and rotation. While performing this active range of motion the patient is asked to report on pain generation (location, quality, radiation, consistency and intensity) with motion.

As for every patient it is important to first rule out infectious, metabolic or metastatic causes of neck pain. This includes visceral pain as abdominal contents can refer pain to the neck.

Magnetic resonance imaging adds diagnostic information; however, due to its relatively high false-negative and false-positive rates, it should be used to confirm diagnosis based on history and physical exam. When cervical discography is performed in accordance with the results of a preprocedural MRI, imaging was found to have a false-positive rate of 51% and a false negative rate of 27%. Therefore, the combination of clinical symptoms, MRI, and discography provides the most information for decision making and can improve the management of cervical discogenic pain.

The preferred treatment for cervical DDD is conservative, such as the McKenzie approach and cervicothoracic stabilization through strengthening programs, combined with aerobic conditioning. The McKenzie method involves extension of the patient's spine in an attempt to "centralize" the pain away from the extremities and more focused on the back, because back pain is generally tolerated better than extremity pain. Treatment emphasizes self-healing exercises rather than passive approaches such as heat, cold or needles. These approaches aim to address the specific mechanical challenges for each patient, i.e. posture and range of motion. Physician or physical therapist recommended exercises and stretches are key to maintaining neck flexibility and releasing stiffness. In addition, over-the-counter (OTC) medications such as NSAIDs or acetaminophen can be useful in reducing inflammation.

Prescription medications such as oral steroids, muscle relaxants or narcotic pain medications may also be used sparingly in dire circumstances and only for acute definable pain. Prolonged narcotic use is ill advised and should only be performed under the direction of a pain specialist.

Surgery for cervical DDD is controversial and should only be considered as a last resort if exhaustive conservative management is not effective. Surgery is often discounted as a treatment option as the natural history of axial neck pain is equivalent to the outcomes of surgical intervention.

Cervical Radiculopathy and Radicular Pain

Sources of neck pain can roughly be grouped into two categories: pain originating from pathology of the soft tissues of the neck, and pain originating from pathology relating to the neurologic elements. Cervical radicular pain and/ or cervical radiculopathy are primarily brought on by pressure on the nerve roots or their blood supply as they exit the spinal column. For clarification, cervical "radicular pain" refers to instances where pain is the only symptom or in referring to the pain itself associated with the patients' pathology. While it is common for patients with cervical radiculopathy to present with pain or have pain as a primary component, cervical "radiculopathy" refers to the conglomeration of symptoms of anesthesia, numbness or hypoesthesia, motor or functional loss, and pain.

Most commonly cervical radiculopathy is brought on by disk degeneration, herniation, and bone spur formation; however any phenomenon leading to pressure, inflammation or irritation, or a compromise to the blood flow of the root or nerve itself can be causative. Disk degeneration occurs with age as the disk loses water content over time, the disk height collapses and subsequently the intervertebral foramen becomes narrowed to the point where it may impinge on the exiting nerves. As little as a 1 mm decrease in disk height can narrow the neuroforamen 29–30%.

Diagnosis begins with a complete history of the patient's symptom onset and progression, followed by physical exam, which includes range of motion testing. Functional reflex testing can implicate specific nerve roots in the pathophysiology of the disease. Absent biceps reflex indicates C5 involvement, whereas a brachioradialis reflex deficit indicates C6 involvement, and a triceps reflex loss corresponding to C7 involvement. Root impingement at C7-T1 has no affected reflex association; impingement on C8 is a highly uncommon source of neck pain. Fatigability is greatly increased in cases of cervical radiculopathy and consequently weakness is more pronounced with repetitive strength testing. Nerve recruitment is impaired when axons within the nerve are compromised by the compressive pathology.

Radiculopathy is a clinical diagnosis. Treatment of radiculopathy is aided by obtaining the appropriate imaging studies. Anterior-posterior, lateral, flexion and extension radiographs of the cervical spine can reveal the location of pressure on nerve roots, brought on by things such as disk degeneration and disk height collapse, degenerative spondylolisthesis, or even the presence of a bone spur. An MRI adds an additional level of treatment guidance by displaying the nerve along its path from the spinal cord through its respective neuroforamen and pinpointing the exact location of compression. It is important to note that MRIs are known to be overly sensitive. The MRI should be used to corroborate a physical exam finding and not for fishing for something to treat.

Though traumatic head or neck injury can rupture the annulus of the disk causing herniation of the disk into the space of the exiting nerves, typically the presenting herniation is degenerative and atraumatic in nature. The narrowing of the neuroforamen and consequent compression of the exiting nerve or nerve root occurs through direct compression from a disk herniation, collapse of the disk height and decrease in cross-sectional area of the foramen, or even through the formation of a disk-osteophyte complex. This compressive complex can cause direct compression of the nerve, nerve root or compression of the vascular supply to the nerve leading to ischemia of the axons within. The end result is essentially the same and the real task becomes first distinguishing cervical radiculopathy or radicular pain from that due to mechanical or axial neck pain. In general, mechanical neck pain stops at the shoulder, rarely traveling down the upper limb, while shooting or burning pain down the upper limb in a predictable dermatomal distribution indicates cervical radiculopathy. When the pain is neurogenic in nature it is often accompanied by tingling, weakness, or reflex abnormalities in the affected limb.

When the picture is not clear through physical exam, history, radiographs and MRI, electrodiagnostic testing can further distinguish cervical radiculopathy from other sources of pain. An electromyogram (EMG) can help to pinpoint the location of the nerve conduction block or compression. Peripheral nerve lesions can coexist with cervical radiculopathy and can make the diagnosis more difficult to elucidate. In the event that cervical radiculopathy is identified by the aforementioned methods, an appropriate and informed nonoperative plan can then be developed between patient and physician. Treatment begins with anti-inflammatory medications and physical therapy. Epidural injections, nerve blocks, and facet injections all have merit and should be directed by a pain management specialist or a surgeon. Ultimately surgery for cervical radiculopathy has a great track record and is an option when conservative treatment is not effective.

Cervical Spondylotic Myelopathy

Cervical spondylotic myelopathy (CSM) is a condition that often develops with age, in which normal wear and tear over the course of several years progressively narrows the spinal canal, causing a variety of symptoms. The slow compression of the spinal cord seen in CSM most commonly presents as a gradual worsening numbness, tingling, weakness, and gait instability accompanied by neck stiffness. The pain component of CSM is generally due to facet arthropathy and alteration of the mechanics of the neck leading to muscle strain and spasm.

Physical and neurological tests are designed to determine the presence of spinal cord dysfunction. If there is pressure on the spinal cord, flexion of the neck may cause an electric shock like sensation (Lhermitte's sign), which may or may not be accompanied by tingling in the hands. Upon reflex examination, a characteristic finding of CSM is hyper-reflexia of the triceps reflex (C7) with an absent biceps and supinator reflex (C5 and C6). Other indications of spinal cord dysfunction that may be present include Hoffman's sign (reflexive contraction of fingers and/or thumb upon a flick of middle finger distal phalanx) and Babinski sign (pathologic extension of big toe upon stroking the sole of the foot). Hyperactive pectoralis reflex (elicited upon striking the pectoralis muscle in the deltopectoral groove) can indicate cord compression between the C2-C4 levels.

The patient should be asked to perform a tandem gait across the examining room. This should be done with the patient looking straight ahead (at the examiner or at a fixed point on the wall) so as to remove visual cues. Myelopathy can have a profound effect on gait with many individuals unable to perform a tandem gait without losing balance. The patient should be asked about hand awkwardness or clumsiness; difficulty manipulating small objects, buttoning shirts or dropping things.

Anterior-posterior, lateral, flexion and extension views of the cervical spine help to elucidate alignment, degenerative spondylosis, and yield a basic understanding of the space available for the cervical spinal cord. When the signs or symptoms are concerning for myelopathy, an MRI is the next step, and is used to evaluate for compression of the spinal cord. Electrodiagnostic testing (EMG) is generally of limited value in the setting of suspected myelopathy and should only be reserved for concomitant radicular complaints.

Neck pain associated with cervical spondylosis in the absence of myelopathy can often find relief through nonsurgical treatment including NSAIDs, physical therapy for neck strengthening and posture control, and isometric neck exercises. Cervical spondylosis in the setting of myelopathy and cord compression is often treated with surgical decompression and fusion in order to prevent progression of myelopathy.

Referred Pain

Referred pain is the general term for pain felt in one area of the body that is caused by activation of nerves from a different area of the body. A classic example is referred left shoulder pain upon irritation of the diaphragm. Pain

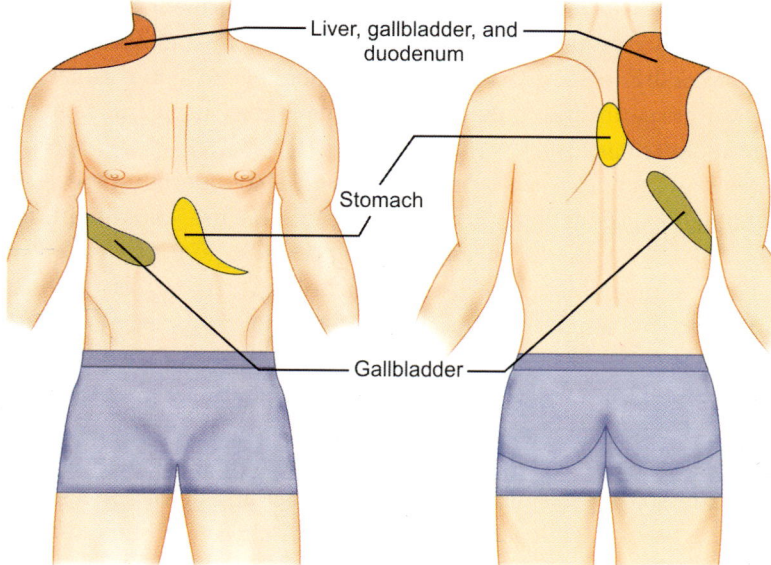

Fig. 8.1: Referred pain and its origin. It can be seen from the drawing that there are various visceral sources of pain that can refer to areas that patients will refer to as neck and/or upper back pain. Based on original drawing by Mounts AM.

fibers supplying the diaphragm enter the spinal cord at the levels C3 to C5, the same level at which pain fibers from the shoulder enter. Upon irritation of the diaphragm as seen in strenuous exercise or from inflammation of a nearby organ, the pain fibers of C3-C5 will send a strong signal to the brain, which is sometimes misinterpreted as pain originating in the shoulder due to the fact that the nerves are entering the spinal cord at the same level (nerve crosstalk). Pathology within the neck can be another source of referred shoulder pain such as seen in cervical spondylosis and disk prolapse. Because of this, a patient presenting with a chief complaint of shoulder pain presents a challenging scenario.

Referred pain to the neck can arise from metabolic, inflammatory or neoplastic pathology originating in the heart, lungs, abdominal viscera, or temporomandibular joint (Fig. 8.1). Myocardial infarction often has a neck pain component; sensory nerve fibers of the heart travel through dorsal roots and ganglia of T1-T4. The T2 dermatome in particular covers the back of the neck and shoulder, while the rest of T1-T4 can project a painful sensation to the left chest and arm in the event of a myocardial infarction. Temporomandibular joint dysfunction is often associated with chronic neck pain and headaches.

Referred pain can originate in multiple areas of the body, and each one will require treatment specific to the area causing the painful stimuli. For this reason, treatment of referred pain must first start with identifying the source of the pain as intrinsic to the area or extrinsically caused by crossing of pain fibers from a remote source. In the case of pain in the neck or shoulder, there are a variety of physical tests that can be performed. The first test however should be visual inspection for bruising, abrasions, or deformity and to ensure the arms and shoulders are bilaterally symmetric. Asymmetry could indicate a shoulder dislocation, atrophy of the serratus anterior muscle, or thoracic scoliosis. After a visual inspection, functional pain is assessed by stimulating the muscle in the area through active assisted, active resisted and passive range of motion modalities, and superficial and deep palpation. If the presenting pain worsens with stimulation of the symptomatic area, it is likely that the pain is not referred. It is important to realize that any physical exam modality has the potential to elicit new pain and this pain must be differentiated from the pain of presentation.

Referred pain does not worsen with movement of the shoulder and arm. Pain in the neck however may worsen with movement of the shoulder and it is imperative that the physician constantly reassesses where exactly the pain is felt upon movement. As an example, the Apley maneuver can be performed to assess shoulder range of motion; having the patient touch the superior aspect of the contralateral scapula with their hand tests abduction and external rotation of the shoulder, while having the patient touch the inferior aspect of the contralateral scapula tests internal rotation and adduction. The anatomy involved in this maneuver includes the glenohumeral joint as well as the scapulothoracic articulation. If pain levels are increased from rest upon performing the Apley maneuver, the patient is more likely suffering from a myogenic condition than from a neurogenic or referred pain source.

If the origin of the pain can be narrowed through one of the aforementioned modalities, radiographic evaluation can be an important aid in determining the extent of the skeletal involvement. It is generally recommended that the existing pain be present for at least 3 weeks without improvement in severity prior to subjecting the patient to a dose of radiation. Pain that is improving or that is atraumatic and acute (less than 3 weeks) in nature is less likely to gain diagnostic accuracy through the addition of an X-ray. Pain that is not able to be elicited with a physical exam and consequently is not localizable to the shoulder and/or the neck, requires further evaluation which may include blood work with or without a chest X-ray, which will provide a clearer picture of any distant source of pain that may be referring to the shoulder. It is also important to remember referent sources of pain and to perform a physical exam of the chest and abdomen in conjunction with your focused musculoskeletal exam, when appropriate.

Red Flags

It is important to remember the spectrum of pathologies that can result in neck pain ranges from infectious, metabolic or metastatic disease, to primary orthopedic issues. As in many areas of medicine there are signs and symptoms that must be recognized early as they may indicate serious underlying pathology. Physicians should be wary of these so-called "red flags" occasionally associated with neck pain and be prepared to react in an expedited manner. After a thorough history and physical examination reveals the presence of the "red flag", a swift execution of a well-designed algorithm will then help the examiner to better weigh the possibility of these conditions. Table 8.1 lists possible "red flags" which may indicate more serious causes of neck pain and the appropriate next step in diagnosis.

PHYSICAL EXAM

Visual Inspection + Subsequent Physical Testing

In the case of pain in the neck or shoulder, there are a variety of physical tests that can be performed. The first test however should be visual inspection for bruising, abrasions, or deformity and to ensure the arms and shoulders are bilaterally symmetric. Asymmetry could indicate a shoulder dislocation, partial weakness of the serratus anterior muscle, or thoracic scoliosis among other pathologies. In assessing active range of motion in flexion, extension and lateral rotation, it is important to remember that "normal" values can vary between men and women, with women having slightly increased range of motion compared to men of the same age, and it can be expected that with each change of 10 years of age, both men and women can be expected to lose 5° of neck extension and 3° of all other ranges of motion (normal ranges of motion included at the end of this section). After a visual inspection, functional pain is assessed by stimulating the muscle in the area through active assisted, active resisted and passive range of motion modalities, and superficial and deep palpation. If the presenting pain worsens with stimulation of the symptomatic area, it is likely that the pain is not referred from another area. It is important to realize that any physical exam modality has the potential to elicit new pain and this pain must be differentiated from the pain of presentation. An easy way to determine the difference between shoulder pain and referred neck pain to the shoulder is that referred pain does not get worse with movement of the shoulder and arm.

Normal Ranges of Cervical Motion

- *Flexion*: 80–90°
- *Extension*: 70°
- *Lateral flexion*: 20–45° on both sides
- *Rotation*: 90° of rotation to both sides.

Table 8.1: The so-called "red flags" of neck pain, the concerning possibility and the appropriate next step in diagnosis/management.

Pain associated with	Concern	Next step
Bilateral upper or bilateral lower extremity neurologic dysfunction (weak/numb/dysesthesia)	Cord level injury or compression Underlying myelopathy Demyelinating disorder	X-ray, MRI of appropriate area (cervical, thoracic, or lumbar)
Gait dysfunction		
Bowel or bladder incontinence		
Sexual dysfunction		
Fumbling of hands—difficulty manipulating small objects		
Burning or electrical sensation down the back and into limbs upon anterior flexion of the neck (Lhermitte's sign)		
Drop attacks, dizziness, upward gaze, vision changes	Vascular insufficiency (e.g. Bow-Hunter's syndrome)	Provocative digital subtraction angiography (DSA)
Constitutional signs/symptoms (fever, chills, night sweats, unintentional weight loss)	Infection, metabolic, metastatic lesion or infiltrative process, pathologic fracture, systemic inflammatory disease	Appropriate workup for the like involving laboratory work and imaging directed by clinical suspicion
Nocturnal pain		
Swollen lymph nodes		
Severe pain that is both consistent and persistent		
History of TB, HIV, cancer or inflammatory arthritis		
Relatively young (< 20 years) or old (> 55 years)		
Significant preceding trauma or previous neck surgery	Fracture, ligamentous injury	ATLS workup (X-ray, CT, etc.)

(TB: Tuberculosis; HIV: Human immunodeficiency virus; ATLS: Advanced Trauma Life Support; CT: Computed tomography).

Additional Exam Maneuvers

Spurling Maneuver

The patient's head is turned toward the affected side and extended while applying gentle downward pressure to the top of the patient's head. The maneuver effectively decreases the size of the neuroforamen. In the setting of a disk herniation and consequent neuroforaminal encroachment, the exiting nerve roots can be further irritated. The test is positive if pain radiates along the corresponding dermatome ipsilaterally.

Apley Maneuver

In some clinical presentations, pain in the neck may worsen with movement of the shoulder and it is imperative that the physician constantly reassesses where exactly the pain is felt upon movement. As an example, the Apley maneuver can be performed to assess shoulder range of motion; having the patient touch the superior aspect of the contralateral scapula with their hand tests abduction and external rotation of the shoulder, while having the patient touch the inferior aspect of the contralateral scapula tests internal rotation and adduction. The anatomy involved in this maneuver includes the glenohumeral joint as well as the scapulothoracic articulation. If pain levels are increased from rest upon performing the Apley maneuver, the patient is more likely suffering from a myogenic condition than from a neurogenic or referred pain source.

Romberg Test

The Romberg test is designed to assess neurological function and proprioception. First, the physician asks the patient to stand with their feet together and eyes closed, with the physician standing close by as a precaution in case the patient falls. With the patient's eyes closed, the physician watches the patient for one full minute, accounting for any movements the patient makes in reference to a fixed object in the room; a positive Romberg sign is noted upon the patient swaying or starting to fall. Positive test indicates a disturbance of either the vestibular (labyrinthine) or sensory (proprioceptive) mechanisms of balance and coordination.

Hoffman's Reflex/Sign

Hoffman's reflex test is used to detect the presence of pathology of the corticospinal tract and/or spinal cord compression. The test is done by flicking or tapping terminal phalanx of the middle or ring finger. A positive response is seen with flexion of the terminal phalanx of the thumb.

Clonus

Clonus is a series of involuntary rhythmic muscle contractions elicited upon reflex testing, that are commonly associated with upper motor neuron lesions. The contractions may or may not be accompanied with spasticity. Clonus can be differentiated from fasciculations (lower motor neuron source) in that clonus tends to be provoked by testing the patient's reflexes; fasciculations are not.

Babinski Sign

The Babinski sign is obtained by stimulating the lateral aspect of the sole of the foot. The examiner begins the stimulation at the heel and goes forward to the base of the toes. Upon stimulation, a positive Babinski sign is elicited if the patient's big toe dorsiflexes and other toes fan out, instead of the normal motion of reflexively plantar flexing. A useful way to attempt to elicit a Babinski response that requires no special equipment is with firm pressure from the examiner's thumb. Although newborn babies commonly exhibit Babinski sign, a positive sign in an older child or adult is abnormal, and is usually a sign of a problem in the pyramidal tract of the central nervous system.

Lhermitte's Sign

This sign is positive when sudden transient electric-like shocks extend down the spine when flexing the head forward. The causes of Lhermitte's sign include multiple sclerosis, cervical spondylosis, herniation of a cervical disk, a cervical spinal cord tumor, and subacute combined degeneration (caused by vitamin B12 deficiency). Shocks radiating up the spine are sometimes referred to as reverse Lhermitte's sign.

Straight Line Gait

Straight line gait or "tandem gait" tests are performed in order to help diagnose ataxia. The test involves having the patient walk in a straight line with the toes of their back foot touching the heels of their front foot on each step. The physician should always walk alongside the patient in the event that the patient starts to fall or lose balance.

CONCLUSION

Neck pain is a very common complaint in the adult population. It is important to always identify any serious underlying cause of neck pain, such as fracture, infection, carcinoma, or referred pain from a visceral organ. In the absence of myelopathy or radiculopathy, the treatment for axial neck pain remains conservative, as surgical interventions can lead to unpredictable results with the added risk of a surgical procedure.

SUGGESTED READING

1. American Academy of Orthopaedic Surgeons. (2015). Cervical Spondylosis (Arthritis of the Neck). [online] Available from http://orthoinfo.aaos.org/topic. cfm?topic=A00369. [Accessed November, 2015].
2. American Academy of Orthopedic Surgeons. (2015). Cervical Radiculopathy (Pinched Nerve). [online] Available from orthoinfo.aaos.org/topic.cfm?topic= A00332. [Accessed November, 2015].
3. Available from now.aapmr.org/msk/disorders-spine/Pages/Cervical-Whiplash. aspx#references. [Accessed November, 2015].
4. Barnsley L, Lord SM, Wallis BJ, et al. The prevalence of chronic cervical zygapophyseal joint pain after whiplash. Spine (Phila Pa 1976). 1995;20(1):20-5; discussion 26.

5. Bastian AJ, Mink JW, Kaufman BA, et al. Posterior vermal split syndrome. Ann Neurol. 1998;44(4):601-10.

6. DePalma AF, Rothman RH, Lewinnek GE, et al. Anterior interbody fusion for severe cervical disc degeneration. Surg Gynecol Obstet. 1972;134(5):755-8.

7. Gore DR, Sepic SB, Gardner GM. Roentgenographic findings of the cervical spine in asymptomatic people. Spine (Phila Pa 1976). 1986;11(6):521-4.

8. Grubb SA, Kelly CK. Cervical discography: clinical implications from 12 years of experience. Spine (Phila Pa 1976). 2000;25(11):1382-9.

9. Houston Methodist. A Patient's Guide to Cervical Radiculopathy. [online] www.methodistorthopedics.com/cervical-radiculopathy. [Accessed November, 2015].

10. MedicineNet.com. Definition of Babinski sign. [online] Available from www.medicinenet.com/script/main/art.asp?articlekey=7186. [Accessed November, 2015].

11. MedicineNet.com. Degenerative Disc Disease and Sciatica. [online] http://www.medicinenet.com/degenerative_disc/article.htm. [Accessed November, 2015].

12. Medterms Medical Dictionary A-Z List. Definition of Lhermitte sign. [online] Available from MedicineNet.com. [Accessed November, 2015].

13. National Institute of Neurological Disorders and Stroke. Neurological diagnostic tests and procedures. [online] Available from www.ninds.nih.gov/disorders/misc/diagnostic_tests.htm. [Accessed November, 2015].

14. Neck Pain Referred to the Shoulder. [online] Available from www.shoulderdoc.co.uk/article.asp?article=1529. [Accessed November, 2015].

15. Radanov BP, Sturzenegger M, Di Stefano G. Long-term outcome after whiplash injury: a 2-year follow-up considering features of injury mechanism and somatic, radiologic, and psychosocial findings. Medicine (Baltimore). 1995;74(5):281-97.

16. Remedy's health.com. Degenerative Disc Disease. [online] Available from www.healthcommunities.com/degenerative-disc-disease/causes-symptoms.shtml. [Accessed November, 2015].

17. Singh AP. Range of Motion of Cervical Spine. [online] Available from bone-andspine.com/range-motion-cervical-spine/. [Accessed November, 2015].

18. The Free Dictionary by Farlex. Babinski reflex. [online] Available from medical-dictionary.thefreedictionary.com/Babinski+reflex. [Accessed November, 2015].

19. Ullrich PF. Cervical Degenerative Disc Disease Treatment Options. [online] Available from www.spine-health.com/conditions/degenerative-disc-disease/cervical-degenerative-disc-disease-treatment-options. [Accessed November, 2015].

20. Ullrich PF. Cervical Stenosis with Myelopathy. [online] Available from www.spine-health.com/conditions/spinal-stenosis/cervical-stenosis-myelopathy. [Accessed November, 2015].

21. United Nations. No WP29-135-17. World Forum for Harmonization of Vehicle Regulations (WP.29), 139th session: United Nations Economic and Social Council. 2005. Request to list in the compendium of candidate global technical regulations (compendium of candidates) the United States of America Federal Motor Vehicle Safety Standard (FMVSS) No. 202—Head restraints; p. 6.

22. WebMD Medical Reference from Healthwise. (2014). Referred Shoulder Pain–Topic Overview. [online] Available from www.webmd.com/pain-management/tc/referred-shoulder-pain-topic-overview. [Accessed November, 2015].

23. Youdas JW, Garrett TR, Suman VJ, et al. Normal range of motion of the cervical spine: an initial goniometric study. Phys Ther. 1992;72(11):770-80.

CHAPTER 9

Headaches

Stephanie Wrobel Goldberg, Alexander J Schupper, Stephen Silberstein

CHIEF COMPLAINT/HISTORY

Headache is one of the most common reasons for visits to the emergency room and out-patient setting. Primary headache (such as migraine and tension-type headache) is a disorder unto itself; no underlying disease process is present. Secondary headache is a manifestation of an underlying disease process.[1] Disorders of the cervical spine and of other structures of the neck have frequently been linked as causes of head pain since many headaches are located in this area.[2]

Healthcare providers need to be aware that neck pain does not have to be of cervical origin. Headaches caused by disorders of the neck can present with different clinical features making it difficult to describe a set of chief complaints to define them. Signs and symptoms on the neurological exam that if present should indicate cervical spine investigation include radicular pain to arms or occipital area, limb weakness, ataxia, upper neuron findings on lower extremities, or hyperactive bladder. Supporting evidence and close temporal relationship of headaches with a cervical disorder is helpful, although ultimately clinical judgment will help establish the diagnosis.

DIFFERENTIAL DIAGNOSIS

The International Classification of Headache Disorders (ICHD) is a detailed hierarchical classification of all headache-related disorders published by the International Headache Society (IHS). This schematic headache classification is divided into three parts, the second one describing headaches attributed to an underlying (secondary) condition. It is under this section of the ICHD that headaches attributed to disorders of cervical structures, including cervicogenic headache are described. Only when a headache occurs for the first time in close temporal relation to a neck disorder should it be considered a secondary headache attributed to that disorder even if it resembles a typical primary headache. There should also be enough supporting evidence that the pain can be attributed to the disorder or lesion.

Box 9.1: Differential diagnosis: secondary headaches.
Trauma to the head and/or neck • Whiplash
Cranial or cervical vascular disorder • Cervical carotid or vertebral artery disorder
Non-vascular intracranial disorder • Low cerebral spinal fluid (CSF) pressure (postdural puncture headache, CSF fistula headache, spontaneous intracranial hypotension)
Headache attributed to disorder of the neck • Cervicogenic headache • Headache attributed to retropharyngeal tendonitis • Headache attributed to craniocervical dystonia
Developmental anomalies of the craniovertebral junction • Headache attributed to Chiari malformation type I

Box 9.1 highlights the headaches linked to cervical spinal causes found in part two of ICHD 3 and further described in detail.[3]

It is important to keep in mind that many other conditions affecting the neck and cervical spine, including infectious process and tumors were not described in this chapter but can certainly lead to head pain.

• *Headache attributed to trauma or injury to the head and/or neck*: When a headache occurs for the first time in close temporal relation to trauma or injury of the head and/or neck, it is considered a secondary headache attributed to the trauma or injury. This is true even when the headache has the characteristics of a primary one. In other words, headache attributed to trauma can present as any type of primary headache as long as it happens in close temporal relation to the trauma. To facilitate the diagnosis the headache must develop within an arbitrary 7-day interval of the trauma or injury. If loss of consciousness is involved, headache should be reported within 7 days after regaining ability to sense or report pain. During the first 3 months it is considered acute; if the headache continues beyond that period it is designated as persistent. Headache may occur as part of a post-concussion syndrome that includes other symptoms such as dizziness, fatigue, psychomotor slowing, decreased concentration, anxiety, irritability, mild memory impairment, insomnia, etc.

Whiplash headache may result from stretch or injury to the upper cervical structures. Some studies suggest that shearing injuries of long axons in the brain stem and upper cord may disrupt central pain and other regulatory mechanisms.[4-8]

Previous history of headache, female gender and presence of comorbid psychiatric conditions can all be considered risk factors for the development of headaches after a trauma. The patient's expectations of headache, litigation issues, sleep disruption and medication overuse can certainly contribute to persistence of pain.

- *Headache attributed to cervical carotid or vertebral artery disorder*: Sudden onset headache and/or pain to the face or neck can be a presentation of cervical or carotid artery dissection. Usually the pain is ipsilateral to the dissected vessel and may be a warning symptom preceding a stroke. Associated ipsilateral Horner's syndrome, painful tinnitus of sudden onset or painful CN XII palsy is highly suggestive of carotid dissection. Diagnosis is based on cervical magnetic resonance imaging (MRI) with fat suppression, carotid Dopplers, magnetic resonance angiography (MRA), computed tomographic angiography (CTA), and in doubtful cases, conventional angiography.
- *Headache attributed to low cerebral spinal fluid (CSF) pressure*: This headache is usually, but not invariably, orthostatic, that is, it significantly worsens soon after sitting upright or standing and improves after lying horizontally. It may be accompanied by neck pain, tinnitus, changes in hearing, photophobia and/or nausea. The most common reason for a low CSF pressure headache is following a lumbar puncture procedure that leaves a leakage through the pierced dura. A dural fistula from trauma to the spine can also lead to the same diagnosis. According to the ICHD 3 beta criteria, postdural puncture headache should develop within 5 days of the procedure. It tends to resolve spontaneously within 2 weeks, or after sealing of the leak with autologous epidural lumbar patch. In patients with typical orthostatic headache and no apparent cause on exam and workup, it is reasonable to empirically provide an autologous lumbar epidural blood patch.
- *Cervicogenic headache*: Rather than a disease entity, cervicogenic headache is thought to be the clinical manifestation of a disorder of the cervical spine and its component bone, disk and/or soft tissue elements, usually, but not invariably, accompanied by neck pain. There should be clinical, laboratory and/or radiological evidence of a disorder or lesion within the cervical spine or soft tissues of the neck capable of causing headaches. Evidence of causation is demonstrated by the presence of at least two of the following: (1) temporal relation to the onset of the cervical disorder or appearance of the lesion; (2) parallel improvement or resolution of headaches with improvement or resolution of cervical disorder; (3) headache is made significantly worse by provocative cervical motion.

  This headache is usually unilateral, beginning in the neck and eventually spreading to the oculofrontotemporal area where the maximum pain is. Pericranial tenderness and radiation of pain from the occipital area to frontal/periorbital regions is suggestive but neither specific or necessary for the diagnosis. Prevalence estimates of cervicogenic headache range from 0.4% to 2.5% of the general population to 15–20% of patients with chronic headaches.[9] The accepted cervical causes of headache include tumors of craniovertebral junction and upper cervical spine, Paget disease of the skull with secondary basilar invagination, osteomyelitis of the upper cervical vertebrae, rheumatoid arthritis of the upper cervical spine, and ankylosing spondylitis of the upper cervical spine.[10] For educational purposes, headaches attributed to trauma to the neck and developmental anomalies will be described separately.

Acquired lesions of the craniovertebral junction and upper cervical spine, such as primary tumors (meningioma, schwannoma, ependymoma), Paget disease of the skull with secondary basilar invagination, osteomyelitis of the upper cervical vertebrae, and multiple myeloma of the skull base or upper cervical vertebrae may produce headache by erosion of pain-sensitive structures or traction of upper cervical nerve roots.[2]

Rheumatoid arthritis of the upper cervical spine produces headaches through a variety of mechanisms including inflammation of the synovial atlanto-occipital and atlanto-axial joints and stretching of upper cervical ligaments and nerve roots caused by atlanto-axial subluxation (may also occur in ankylosing spondylitis).

The presence of cervical spondylosis and/or cervical disk disease should not necessarily be taken as the cause of a patient's headaches. Their almost ubiquitous existence in people over 40 years old makes it difficult to establish causality or even strong association.[2]

- *Headache attributed to retropharyngeal tendonitis*: Retropharyngeal tendonitis, also called retropharyngeal calcific tendonitis (RCT), is a common form of calcific periarthritis in the tendon of the longus colli muscle.[11] IHS criteria for headache attributed to retropharyngeal tendonitis include unilateral or bilateral non-pulsating pain in the back of the neck, radiating to the back of the head or to the whole head.[3]

The radiologic diagnosis can be made from finding enlargement of the retropharyngeal space due to fluid collection, and subsequently from calcifications present in the superior longus colli tendons. RCT may occasionally mimic a retropharyngeal abscess (RPA), presenting with symptoms of sore throat, low-grade fever, mild leukocytosis and elevated sedimentation rate.

Headache is caused by inflammation or calcification of retropharyngeal soft tissues, and aggravated severely by extension of the neck, rotation of the head and/or swallowing.

In a literature review of 71 case reports of patients with RCT, the most common symptom was neck pain (94%), followed by limited range of motion (45%).[12] Upper carotid dissection should be ruled out.

- *Headache attributed to craniocervical dystonia*: Dystonia is a neuromuscular disorder defined as continuous muscle contractions that lead to repetitive movements and abnormal posturing. Craniocervical dystonia affects muscles of the neck innervated by the cranial nerves. Pain is thought to originate from muscle hyperactivity and persistent contraction as well as secondary changes in sensitization.

Within the nervous system, craniocervical dystonia is thought to originate from abnormality of the basal ganglia-thalamo-cortical circuitry[13] as well as from chemical imbalances of the gamma-aminobutyric acid (GABA)-releasing cerebellar Purkinje cells, particularly due to dysfunction of the Na^+/K^+ pump.[14]

Headache attributed to craniocervical dystonia should develop in close temporal relation to the onset of the craniocervical dystonia or there should be clinical signs that implicate a source of pain in the hyperactive muscle (e.g. pain is precipitated or exacerbated by muscle contraction, movements, sustained posture, or external pressure). Both conditions are expected to worsen in parallel and pain should improve or resolve upon treatment of the abnormal movements.[3]

- *Developmental anomalies of the craniovertebral junction and upper cervical spine*: Developmental anomalies of the craniovertebral junction and upper cervical spine frequently cause headaches.[15] More than 3 decades ago, headache was reported as the presenting complaint in a quarter of patients with anomalies such as basilar invagination, congenital atlanto-axial dislocation, or separate odontoid.[16] With the advent of MRI, we now know that most of these patients also have soft tissue anomalies, such as Chiari type I malformation.[17]

    Chiari malformation type I, also known as Arnold-Chiari malformation, is a malformation of the brain consisting of a downward displacement of the cerebellar tonsils through the foramen magnum. As the cerebellar tonsils descend, the subarachnoid space at the craniocervical junction can be compressed leading to obstruction of CSF outflow. Headache is usually occipital or suboccipital, of short duration (less than 5 minutes) and provoked by cough or other Valsalva-like maneuver. It may be associated with other neurological symptoms and/or clinical signs, especially when a cervical spinal cord syrinx is present. The official diagnosis requires at least a 5-mm caudal displacement of the cerebellar tonsils on an MRI of the brain. Often this is an incidental finding in an otherwise asymptomatic patient and so far there have been no studies proving correlation between severity of headache and extent of herniation.[2]

ANATOMY AND PATHOPHYSIOLOGY

Pain sensation from the front of the head and face as well as anterior skull contents, is mainly carried by the three divisions of the trigeminal nerve [cranial nerve (CN) V]: ophthalmic, maxillary and mandibular. Below the tentorium there is more complex innervation with contribution from the facial nerve (CN VII), glossopharyngeal nerve (CN IX), vagal nerve (CN X) as well as the C2 and C3 nerve roots.[18]

Upper cervical roots, primarily C2 and C3, carry pain sensation from posterior portions of the head as well as the dura in the posterior fossa. C1 is essentially a motor nerve innervating several suboccipital muscles. Lesions or dysfunction of these nerves may produce pain localized to the innervated area[19] and are often referred to different areas given the overlap of central pathways.

The bony and ligamentous anatomy of the upper cervical spine and its articulation with the base of the skull is complex.[12] Deformity or dysfunction in these areas is often to blame for head pain. Nociceptive cervical structures include joints, periosteum, ligaments of the cervical spine, muscles around the cervical spine, cervical roots, nerves and arteries.[2]

Over the last 15 years there have been advances in the genetics of migraine as well as some very novel ideas about a brainstem "migraine integrator" that provide a pathophysiologic explanation of migraine and headache in general. Both the trigeminal and upper cervical spinal root synapse in the dorsal horn region of the upper cervical cord, a portion of which contains the spinal trigeminal nucleus (STN). These two systems are intermixed, which explains the often complex pain referral patterns seen in pain conditions of the head, face, and upper neck. Interestingly, afferents of CN IX and X and the sensory roots of CN VII also run in the spinal tract of the trigeminal nerve and synapse in the STN.[18]

Referred pain to the back of the head from cervical structures can also be mediated by the greater and lesser occipital nerves, extensions of C2 sensory roots. There is no known physiologic basis for cephalic referral of pain originating from cervical segments below C4.[2] Referred pain is thought

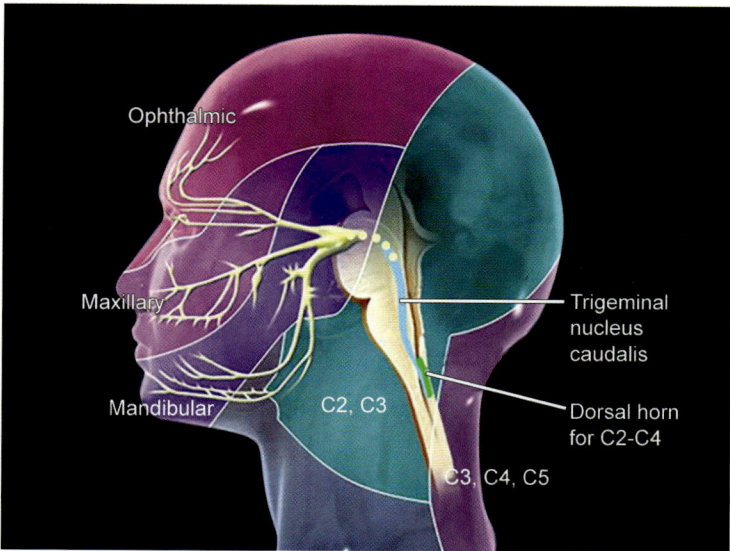

Fig. 9.1: Distribution of pain from the three divisions of the trigeminal nerve and the upper cervical nerves.
Courtesy: Dr Stasha Gominak, MD. Sleep, Chronic Pain, and Headaches website.

to be due to convergence of multiple first-order afferents on wide dynamic range neurons, leading to false or mixed localization. Referral patterns in the head, face and neck can include any site innervated by CN V, VII, IX and X as well as C2 and C3 (Fig. 9.1).[18]

PHYSICAL EXAM AND WORKUP

Performing an expensive battery of exams on all patients with headache is neither cost-effective nor appropriate. But, failure to perform diagnostic tests in certain patients however may result in missing life-threatening, yet treatable conditions.[1]

In addition to obtaining a thorough history and physical exam, the clinician should be attentive to signs and symptoms suggestive of secondary headaches. An easy mnemonic SNOOPP can be used as a reminder of the most important ones: "S" for systemic signs and symptoms. The presence of fever and meningismus should be concerning for meningitis. An underlying history of cancer should require investigations for intracerebral metastatic disease. "N" for neurological signs and symptoms. Any focal neurological complaint or finding on exam, especially if persistent should raise concerns. "O" for onset. Abrupt onset headaches can be a clinical presentation of ruptured aneurysm and subarachnoid hemorrhage. New onset of headaches after the age of 50 in a patient with no underlying history of headaches requires further investigation. "P" for pattern change and postural component. Any changes in frequency or quality of primary headaches can be suggestive of development of a secondary concomitant condition. Headaches that are influenced by vertical versus horizontal position may suggest intracranial hyper or hypotension (Table 9.1).

In particular cases MRI of the cervical spine and electromyography/nerve conduction studies may be necessary for further evaluation. Computed tomography (CT) myelography or CSF flow MRI can be performed if there is suspicion of altered spinal cerebral fluid pressure.

Table 9.1: Red flags.

S	Systemic signs and symptoms	e.g. Fever, weight loss, history of malignancy, HIV
N	Neurological signs and symptoms	e.g. Papilledema, sensory, motor, diplopia, bulbar, meningismus
O	Onset	e.g. Abrupt vs. gradual
O	Older than 50 years	e.g. Patients older than 50 years
P	Pattern change	e.g. Change in frequency or quality of underlying headache
P	Postural component	e.g. Intracranial hypotension or hypertension

TREATMENT

The management of headaches attributed to disorders of the neck will depend on its underlying cause. In general, pharmacologic treatment with analgesics, anti-inflammatories and muscle relaxants may provide short-lived benefit but long-term use is precluded by side effects. Small, noncontrolled case series have reported moderate success with nerve block injections which can be used diagnostically as well as therapeutically. Blockade of the C2 roots or greater occipital nerve tend to provide some relief with lower side effects.[20]

Rarely, well-selected patients in a precarious situation nonresponsive to other treatment options, may benefit from more invasive procedures such as decompression of the spinal dura followed by stabilization and fusion.[21] Jansen et al. published a series of 28 patients with bilateral cervicogenic headache submitted to the above mentioned procedure followed in a prospective fashion. Among the 28 patients, 9 reported pain freedom after 5 months of follow-up. Even though the numbers seem promising, the placebo response to surgical intervention is very high and its use in treating cervicogenic headache requires controlled studies. Other procedures are listed in Box 9.2.[22] Physiotherapy, relaxation techniques and psychotherapy are other modalities that can be selectively considered.

In a randomized double-blind, placebo-controlled crossover study by Linde et al. 28 adult patients with a long-standing and treatment-resistant cervicogenic headaches were treated with injections of either onabotulinum toxin A or placebo given in fixed sites in the neck muscles on the painful side. There were no significant differences favoring the use of onabotulinum toxin A in neck muscles in cervicogenic headache.[23] However, onabotulinum toxin A is effective in chronic migraine with neck pain.[24]

The consensus in the treatment of cervical and carotid artery dissection favors the use of heparin followed by warfarin for 3–6 months according to the quality of arterial recovery.

Patients with Chiari I malformations who have minimal or equivocal symptoms without syringomyelia can be treated conservatively. Mild neck pain and headaches can be treated with analgesics, muscle relaxants, and occasional use of a soft collar. Frankly symptomatic patients should be offered

Box 9.2: Invasive procedures for cervicogenic headache.
• Nerve blocks
• Cryoanalgesia
• Radiofrequency procedure
• Operative procedure
• Electrical stimulation

Note: With permission from Fredriksen TA. (2008).[20]

surgical treatment aiming to decompress the cervicomedullary junction and restore normal CSF flow in the region of foramen magnum.

Currently, treatment options for dystonia include physical, medicinal, and surgical intervention. Occupational therapies can be used to improve daily living activities such as swallowing or speaking (i.e. in the case of lingual or laryngeal dystonia). Anticholinergics can be administered to limit hyperactivity in the muscles. Local injections of botulinum toxin have brought a dramatic improvement in this condition, with a success rate in more than two-thirds of patients with segmental dystonia.[25]

In severe cases, surgical interventions such as deep brain stimulation (DBS) surgery have proven effective[26] and work by altering the stimulation of the basal ganglia circuitry. By improving the pain and pressure of the muscles caused by the craniocervical dystonia, the subsequent headache should presumably subside.

Retropharyngeal tendonitis is managed with nonsteroidal anti-inflammatory medications. Surgical drainage may be attempted, but is difficult and often not needed.[27] Additionally, steroids may be prescribed, as well as opiate analgesics while the pain is present.[12] These therapies are prescribed to decrease the inflammation and retropharyngeal space, leading to a decrease in neck pain and pressure, and subsequent headache.

CONCLUSION

Disorders of the cervical spine and of other structures of the neck can cause head pain. The overlapping pathways between the trigeminal system and upper cervical roots offer the anatomical and pathophysiological basis of referred pain from the neck to the head. A close temporal relation to a neck disorder and a headache is usually necessary to establish causality although healthcare providers should be aware that both conditions can happen concomitantly without association to each other. Ideally, an appropriate history and physical exam should guide the diagnosis, limiting expensive tests and invasive procedures to the patients that truly require them. Ultimately, the management of headaches attributed to disorders of the neck will depend on its underlying cause.

REFERENCES

1. Gordon DL. Approach to the patient with acute headache. In: Biller J (Ed). Practical Neurology, 3rd edition. Philadelphia: Lippincott Williams & Wilkins; 2009. pp. 233-48.
2. Göbel H, Edmeads JG. Disorder of the Skull and Cervical Spine. In: Olesen J, Goadsby PJ, Ramadan NM, Tfelt-Hansen P, Welch KM. The Headaches, 3rd edition. Philadelphia: Lippincott Williams & Wilkins; 2006. pp. 1003-12.
3. Headache Classification Subcommittee of the International Headache Society. The International Classification of Headache Disorders, 3rd edition (beta version). Cephalalgia. Cephalalgia. 2013;33(9):629-808.

4. Berry H. Psychological aspects of chronic neck pain following hyperexten-sion-flexion starins of the neck. In: Morley TP (Ed). Current controversies in Neurosurgery. Philadelphia: WB Saunders; 1976. pp. 51-61.
5. Hawkins GW. Flexion and extension injuries of the cervicocapital joints. Clin Orthop. 1962;24:22-33.
6. Vincent MB, Luna RA. Cervicogenic Headache: a comparison with migraine and tension-type headache. Cephalalgia. 1999;19[suppl 25]:11-6.
7. Weiss HD, Stern BJ, Goldberg J. Post-traumatic migraine: chronic migraine precipitated by minor head or neck trauma. Headache. 1991;31(7):451-6.
8. Zwart JA. Neck mobility in different headache disorders. Headache. 1997;37(1): 6-11.
9. Haldeman S, Dagenais S. Cervicogenic headaches: a critical review. Spine J. 2001;1(1):31-46.
10. Göbel H, Heinze A, Kuhn K, et al. Headaches associated with diseases of skull and neck. Schmerz. 1999;13(2):138-50.
11. Kaplan MJ, Eavey RD. Calcific tendinitis of the longus colli muscle. Ann Otol Rhinol Laryngol. 1984;93(3):215-9.
12. Park R, Halpert DE, Baer A, et al. Retropharyngeal calcific tendinitis: case report and review of the literature. Semin Arthritis Rheum. 2010;39(6):504-9.
13. Colosimo C. Craniocerivcal dystonia: clinical and pathophysiological features. Eur J Neurol. 2010;17(1):15-21.
14. Calderon DP, Fremont R, Kraenzlin F, et al. The neural substrates of rapid-onset Dystonia-Parkinsonism. Nat Neurosci. 2011;14(3):357-65.
15. McRae DL. Bony abnormalities at the craniospinal junction. Clin Neurosurg. 1969;16:356-75.
16. Edmeads J. The cervical spine and headache. Neurology. 1988;38(12):1874-8.
17. Pascual J, Oterino A, Berciano J. Headache in type I Chiari malformation. Neurology. 1992;42(8):1519-21.
18. Levin M. Head Pain Anatomy and Physiology. Comprehensive Review of Headache Medicine. New York: Oxford University Press; 2008. pp. 3-20.
19. Farooq K, Williams P. Headache and chronic facial pain. Contin Educ Anaesth Crit Care Pain. 2008;8(4):138-42.
20. Fredriksen TA. Cervicogenic headache: invasive procedures. Cephalalgia. 2008;28 suppl 1:39-40.
21. Jansen J. Surgical treatment of cervicogenic headache. Cephalalgia. 2008;28 (Suppl 1):41-4.
22. Jansen J, Sjaastad O. Cervicogenic headache. Smith/Robinson approach in bilateral cases. Funct Neurol. 2006;21(4):205-10.
23. Linde M, Hagen K, Salvesen O, et al. Onabotulinum toxin A treatment of cer-vicogenic headache: A randomised, double-blind, placebo-controlled cross-over study. Cephalalgia. 2011;31(7):797-807.
24. Dodick DW, Turkel CC, DeGryse RE, et al. Onabotulinum toxin A for treat-ment of chronic migraine: pooled results from the double-blind, random-ized, placebo-controlled phases of the PREEMPT clinical program. Headache. 2010;50(6):921-36.
25. Adam OR, Jankovic J. Treatment of dystonia. Parkinsonism Relat Disord. 2007;13 (Suppl 3):S362-8.
26. Bittar RG1, Yianni J, Wang S, et al. Deep brain stimulation for generalized dystonia and spasmodic torticollis. J Clin Neurosci. 2005;12(1):12-6.
27. Eastwood JD, Hudgins PA, Malone D. Retropharyngeal effusion in acute cal-cific prevertebral tendinitis: diagnosis with CT and MR imaging. AJNR Am J Neuroradiol. 1998;19(9):1789-92.

CHAPTER 10

Gait Abnormalities

Colin Vroome, Christopher M Maulucci, George M Ghobrial, James S Harrop

INTRODUCTION

Walking disability is a common presenting symptom in a variety of clinical settings and to a myriad of different medical specialists. The prevalence of gait abnormalities increases with age, from 15% at age 64 to 40% at age 85.[1] The most common complaints encountered by general practitioners, orthopedic surgeons, neurosurgeons, and neurologists are gait disturbances due to arthritis and radiculopathy.[2] Patients with gait abnormalities commonly present with self-reported joint pain or stiffness, back or neck pain, dizziness, numbness in the feet, weakness, fatigue, muscle pain or cramping, or visual impairment.[2-4]

The history of the patient with a gait disturbance varies widely due to the various etiologies. The duration of the illness may be acute or chronic. Further, symptoms may be episodic or continuous. Exacerbating factors can include medications or environmental conditions. Accompanying symptoms should also be elicited in the history and may include pain, weakness, paresthesias, anxiety about falling, or dizziness.

Gait disorders may also be associated with immobility and falls, both of which contribute to a decline in functional status.[1,2] Whether falls are isolated or recurrent, and the nature of the fall can provide insight into the etiology of the gait disturbance.[2] While gait abnormality is not a common chief complaint of patients presenting to orthopedic surgeons, it is a common secondary symptom.[1] Orthopedic surgeons commonly encounter injuries that occur secondary to falls and identification of gait disorders in these patients may facilitate a multidisciplinary approach to their care.[1]

DIFFERENTIAL DIAGNOSES

Common causes of gait disorders can be divided into musculoskeletal disorders, neurologic disorders, and combined musculoskeletal and neurologic disorders.[1] Patients with degenerative joint disease and those with a prior

---

Box 10.1: Causes of gait abnormalities.

Musculoskeletal disorders
- Antalgic gait
- Trendelenburg gait
- Hip abnormalities
- Knee abnormalities

Myopathies
- Muscular dystrophy
- Duchenne muscular dystrophy
- Becker muscular dystrophy
- Limb girdle muscular dystrophy

Spine related
- Cervical spondylotic myelopathy
- Lumbar spinal stenosis

Lumbar radiculopathy
Sciatica
Peripheral neuropathies
- Metabolic (uremia, diabetes, alcohol)
- Guillain-Barré syndrome
- Chronic inflammatory demyelinating polyradiculoneuropathy
- Charcot-Marie-Tooth disease
- Toxic neuropathies
- Myasthenia gravis
- Lambert-Eaton syndrome

Central nervous dysfunction
- Alzheimer's disease
- Normal pressure hydrocephalus
- Binswanger's disease
- Cerebrovascular accident
- Parkinson's disease
- Drug-induced Parkinsonism
- Progressive supranuclear palsy
- Amyotrophic lateral sclerosis (ALS)
- Multiple sclerosis
- Cerebral palsy
- Dystonia
- Stiff person syndrome
- Microvascular leukoencephalopathy

---

history of orthopedic surgery are the most common patients presenting to general practitioners with gait abnormalities.[3] Gait disorders secondary to stroke, cervical spondylotic myelopathy (CSM), Parkinson's disease (PD), and cerebellar degeneration are also common[1] (Box 10.1).

Musculoskeletal Disorders

Common gait disturbances caused by musculoskeletal disorders include antalgic gait, Trendelenburg gait, and gait disturbances due to hip or knee range of motion abnormalities.[1] Other possible causes of gait abnormalities due to musculoskeletal disorders include postural abnormalities and myopathies. A more detailed discussion of each of these gait patterns and their etiologies are described later in the chapter.

Myopathies

Myopathies may affect gait and have a broad differential diagnosis of their own. Duchenne muscular dystrophy (DMD), Becker muscular dystrophy, and limb girdle muscular dystrophy all cause lower extremity weakness, with DMD typically presenting when children begin to walk; however the latter two often do not present until adulthood.[4] Myotonic muscular dystrophy primarily affects distal muscles, whereas proximal myotonic myopathy affects the proximal leg muscles.[4] Myopathy may be inflammatory, including diagnoses such as dermatomyositis and polymyositis, both presenting with proximal muscle weakness. Inclusion body myositis, another inflammatory myopathy, involves both proximal and distal muscles.[4] Metabolic myopathies that could present with muscle cramps or weakness include McArdle disease and Pompe disease.[4]

Spine Related

Gait disturbances due to combined neurologic and musculoskeletal disorders include myelopathy, and lumbar spinal stenosis.[1] Spondylotic myelopathy occurs due to compression of the spinal cord by osteophytes and ligamentous hypertrophy and is one of the most common causes of gait disturbance in the elderly.[1,2] It occurs most often in the cervical spine, but may occur in the thoracic spine as well. Cervical spondylotic myelopathy may present with neck pain, upper extremity weakness or paresthesias, gait disturbance, and, in severe cases, changes in bladder function.[1,2] The stooped gait of lumbar spinal stenosis occurs due to hypertrophied facets and ligamentum flavum with compression of the cauda equina. Patients may present with a long history of back pain and progression to neurogenic claudication (pain and weakness in the legs when standing and walking, relieved by sitting down or flexing forward).[1]

Radiculopathy and Neuropathy

Causes of a steppage gait (foot drop) include lumbar radiculopathy, sciatica or peripheral neuropathy, and acquired or hereditary peripheral neuropathy.[1] The differential diagnosis for peripheral neuropathies includes metabolic neuropathies due to uremia, diabetes, or alcohol, as well as Guillain-Barré syndrome, chronic inflammatory demyelinating polyradiculoneuropathy (CIDP), Charcot-Marie-Tooth (CMT) disease, and toxic neuropathies (vincristine is one medication known for causing motor neuropathy).[4] Neuromuscular junction disorders may also manifest with gait abnormalities and include myasthenia gravis and Lambert-Eaton syndrome.[5]

Central Nervous Dysfunction

Gait disorders due to central nervous dysfunction in the absence of neural compression include frontal gait, spastic hemiparetic gait, parkinsonian gait, and cerebellar and sensory ataxic gaits.[1] A frontal gait is a characteristically wide-based shuffle which can be caused by Alzheimer's disease, normal-pressure hydrocephalus (NPH), and Binswanger's disease (subcortical dementia). Urinary urgency or incontinence may be more indicative of NPH or Binswanger's disease.[2] A cerebrovascular accident (CVA) due to a hemorrhagic or ischemic lesion along the corticospinal track can cause a spastic hemiparetic gait with recurrent tripping.[1,2] A parkinsonian gait has a characteristic flexed posture and shuffling gait with difficulty initiating ambulation. It can be seen with PD (insidious onset), drug-induced parkinsonism (temporally related to medications), and progressive supranuclear palsy (PSP). A cerebellar ataxic gait is an unsteady gait with a tendency to fall that most commonly occurs with alcoholism (gait abnormality may present without dysarthria or nystagmus), but may also be due to phenytoin toxicity, hereditary ataxias, paraneoplastic syndromes, or vitamin E deficiency. A sensory ataxic gait most commonly occurs due to diabetes with polyneuropathy and combined deficits in vision, proprioception, and vestibular function. Other causes of sensory ataxic gait include tabes dorsalis, vitamin B12 deficiency, and polyneuropathy due to human immunodeficiency virus (HIV) or neurotoxic medications (isoniazid, cisplatin). Additional neurologic disorders causing gait disturbance include orthostatic tremor or myoclonus, neurogenic claudication, amyotrophic lateral sclerosis (ALS), multiple sclerosis (MS), cerebral palsy, dystonia, stiff person syndrome, and microvascular leukoencephalopathy.[5] More rare, hereditary causes that present in childhood include Friedreich's ataxia, spinocerebellar ataxias, and spinal muscular atrophy.[4]

WORKUP

Normal Gait Cycle

The normal gait cycle should first be considered when evaluating a patient with a gait abnormality. The gait cycle is composed of the stance phase (60% of the cycle, beginning with heel strike and ending with toe-lift) and the swing phase (40% of the cycle).[1] A full gait cycle begins when one foot strikes the ground and ends when the same foot strikes the ground.[1] The stance phase includes contraction of the ipsilateral gluteus maximus (to prevent hip flexion), quadriceps (to maintain knee extension), and gluteus medius and minimus to stabilize the ipsilateral hip and elevate the contralateral hip to prepare for swing phase.[5] The swing phase begins when one foot is raised and hip flexion, knee flexion, and ankle dorsiflexion are used to clear the ankle of the ground.[1,5] Swing phase ends when the heel strikes the floor followed by the sole and toes.[1] During the swing phase, the contralateral arm should swing with the elbow slightly flexed (approximately 15°), the forearm should be in midposition, and shoulder slightly is abducted.[5] A period of double limb support accounts for about 10% of the cycle.[1] The pelvis remains relatively level during the cycle with only a slight rise and fall with each step and a slight side-to-side movement due to the displacement of the center of gravity over the weight-bearing side.[1]

Physical Exam

Physical exam should begin with observation of the patient. This starts when the patient enters the office or the room.[1,5] A formal gait examination in the room should begin with the patient sitting.[1,5] The patient should be observed rising from the chair; the ease of this transition and standing posture should be noted.[1] Facial expression should also be observed throughout the exam, noting hypomimia (lack of facial expression common in PD), grimacing (musculoskeletal pain), or fear (secondary to perceived fall risk).[5]

A normal erect posture has a line of gravity, defined as the center of gravity to the ground, of 3–8 cm anterior to the ankles[3] (Fig. 10.1). Optimal posture balances the distribution of body mass around the center of gravity where the compression forces on spinal disks are balanced by the posterior ligamentous tension band allowing for minimal energy expenditure by postural muscles.[1] Signs of asymmetries in posture include head tilt, uneven shoulders or pelvis, scoliosis, or abnormal spine curvature in any plane.[1] A flexed posture may represent PD with cervical dystonia, proprioceptive loss requiring the patient to look at the ground, lumbar spinal stenosis, rigid spinal deformity, or neck extensor weakness due to a neuromuscular disorder.[2,3] A rigid posture may be indicative of kyphosis causing excessive truncal flexion and can be distinguished by its persistence when the patient lays supine.[2,3] Camptocormia, however, is a flexed posture that abates when lying down, and may be due to parkinsonism, dystonia, ALS, or paravertebral myopathies.[3] Leg length discrepancy is another possible cause of gait dysfunction and signs include a dropped shoulder, abducted arm swing, higher pelvis, leg circumduction, and excessive knee flexion on the longer side, and toe out on the shorter side.[1]

With regard to posture, the patient should be examined sitting, supine, and standing.[6] Supine exam allows for the assessment of rigid thoracic or cervical deformities, as well as hip flexion contractures.[6] A sitting exam eliminates the influence of leg length discrepancy and hip flexion contractures in order to assess for thoracic or lumbar abnormalities.[6] Standing provides an assessment of overall sagittal and coronal balance. Flexion, extension, and side bending motions may be used to assess for spinal rigidity and rib hump deformities.[6]

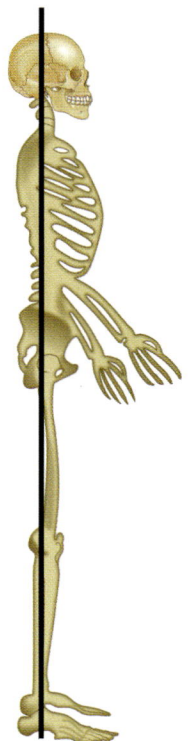

Fig. 10.1: Line depicting the center of gravity.

The base of the patient's stance should be noted, as a wide-based stance may be a sign of imbalance associated with cerebellar ataxia, frontal lobe disease, or myelopathy.[2] More subtle impairment in balance can be elicited by single-limb stance.[2] Romberg's test can also be performed at this time, having the patient close their eyes while standing with the feet together.[2] A positive Romberg's sign is when eye closure causes stance instability; this may be present in sensory ataxia with proprioceptive loss.[2] Stance stability is not affected by eye closure in the case of cerebellar ataxia, an important distinction.[2]

After evaluation of station, the patient should be observed walking at a comfortable pace. A thorough gait exam should include observation of the patient from the front, side, and back.[2,3] First the overall pattern of body movement should be noted followed by individual observation of the lower extremities, torso and upper extremities to distinguish focal problems from general movement disorders.[2] Walking velocity (distance per time), cadence (steps per time), step width, step length (half a gait cycle), and stride length (full gait cycle) are important.[2,3,7] Symmetry of arm swing and use of assistive devices should also be noted.[2,3,7] Asking the patient to walk at a faster pace may elicit more subtle gait abnormalities.[2] Timed tests are also useful for longitudinal assessment of patients; the timed "get up-and-go" test can be performed by timing how long it takes a patient to rise from a seated position, walk 3 m, turn around, walk back to the chair, and sit down.[7] In addition to gait assessment, a complete motor and sensory examination should be conducted. This consists of assessment of the strength of all muscle groups of the upper and lower extremities. Next, testing of light touch and pinprick sensation should be conducted for all dermatomes. An assessment of upper and lower extremity proprioception may follow. To complete the exam, testing of deep tendon reflexes should be performed. This part of the examination is important as a motor weakness or focal sensory dysfunction may be at the root of the gait disturbance.

Some typical gait apraxias should be known as they may help in producing a diagnosis. Difficulty initiating the first step may be a sign of PD or of frontal lobe disease.[2] Patients with PD also may turn "en bloc", turning with the entire body and requiring several steps to do so. A freezing gait may occur when a patient turns, goes through a narrow space, or is anxious, and is characterized by stutter steps that may improve with visual and auditory cuing.[3] This type of gait apraxia may be due to NPH, severe microvascular leukencephalopathy, or PSP.[3]

The stance phase may be affected in multiple ways, possibly by an antalgic gait. In the antalgic gait, lower extremity pain causes the patient to hold the affected limb stiffly (decreasing the range of motion of the ankle, knee, or hip joints) and place his or her body weight gingerly on the limb followed quickly by swinging the unaffected leg forward to minimize the length of the stance phase.[2,3,5] This is accompanied by decreased walking velocity with shortened step length but typically normal cadence.[2] The site of pain should be identified and evaluated for point tenderness, passive and active range of motion, and strength testing. Patellofemoral pain is a common reason for patients to present to practitioners with anterior knee pain characterized by insidious onset and exacerbation by stair climbing or running.[1]

A Trendelenburg gait is also characterized by stance phase abnormalities. It occurs secondary to severe hip abductor insufficiency.[2] During this gait pattern, the contralateral hemipelvis drops during the stance phase of the affected side and greater knee flexion is required to clear the foot during the swing phase[2] (Fig. 10.2). A Trendelenburg gait is dynamic, but a static Trendelenburg test can be performed by first noting the level of the posterior superior iliac spines in double limb stance, then asking the patient to stand on one leg; the test is positive if the hemipelvis contralateral to the stance limb drops.[2]

Inadequate knee extension due to knee flexion contracture can also cause stance phase abnormalities.[2] The flexed knee during stance phase

Normal   Abnormal

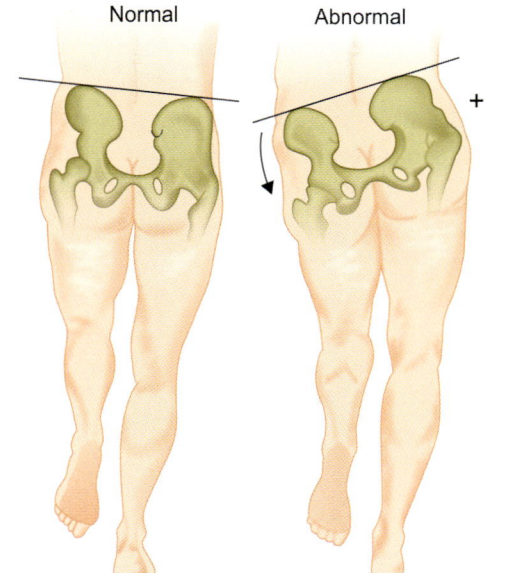

Fig. 10.2: In a Trendelenburg gait pattern, the contralateral hemipelvis drops during the stance phase of the affected side + : Affected hip.

places the body behind the foot resulting in compensatory increased ankle dorsiflexion and premature heel rise to allow the body to align over the foot during midstance.[2] Further musculoskeletal exam of passive and active range of motion of the knee reveals a decreased range of motion at the knee.

A hip flexion contracture causes an inadequate hip extension gait with reduced stride length and duration of single limb support during gait due to prevention of the body from advancing over the supporting foot.[2] Compensatory mechanisms include increased lumbar lordosis, anterior pelvic tilt, and posterior trunk tilt.[2] A cane or walker is typically required for external support, although some patients may adequately compensate with knee flexion and a crouched gait (which may result in concomitant knee flexion contractures and early ambulation fatigue).[2]

The differential diagnosis for swing phase abnormalities is broad, including spastic hemiparetic gait, neurogenic claudication, myelopathy, steppage gait, parkinsonian gait, frontal lobe gait, ataxic gaits, and knee extension or hip flexion contractures.[2,3]

A spastic hemiparetic gait occurs due to lesions of the corticospinal tract such as stroke or MS that result in unilateral circumduction of the advancing leg with audible "scuffing" of the toe.[2,3,5] The affected arm is adducted at the shoulder, and flexed at the elbow, wrist, and fingers, with decreased arm swing.[2] Spasticity causes difficulty with hip and knee flexion and ankle dorsiflexion, requiring circumduction and rocking of the body to the contralateral side to clear the affected limb.[2] A symmetric spastic gait may produce a scissor gait, secondary to excessive thigh adduction and can occur secondary to acquired myelopathy or cerebral palsy with spastic diplegia.

Myelopathic gait disturbance may occur due to cervical or thoracic spine pathology, vitamin B12 deficiency, or MS.[2] Compression of the cervical spinal cord in CSM causes a lower motor nerve lesion at the level of the compression and upper motor nerve dysfunction below the affected level.[2] The lower motor lesions can result in numbness, paresthesias, and loss of fine motor control in the upper extremities.[2] The upper motor neuron lesion results in proximal lower extremity weakness with loss of position and vibration sense due to dorsal column dysfunction.[2] CSM can also present with a spastic paraparetic gait.[2] This gait pattern is characterized by slow and stiff movements at the hip and knee, reduced knee flexion and spastic plantar flexion with reduced toe clearance and compensatory circumduction, decreased step length and walking speed, and increase in step width and time of double limb support.[2] In severe cases, changes in bowel and bladder function may occur.[2] Other causes of myelopathic gait patterns include thoracic disk herniation or MS, as well as vitamin B12 deficiency.[2] A thorough history and neurologic exam to localize the lesion, imaging, and labs can help to differentiate between these etiologies.

A stooped gait secondary to neurogenic claudication can occur due to lumbosacral spinal stenosis and should be considered in patients complaining of leg fatigue.[3] Patients tend to assume a "simian" posture with their shoulders translated anterior to the pelvis.[2] Patients walk slowly in a stooped gait with decreased velocity, shortened stride, and lumbar spine flexed forward. This gait pattern usually is present even before the onset of lower extremity pain.[2] Neurogenic claudication characteristically improves with flexion in an attempt to decrease pressure upon the nerve roots via foraminal widening.[2,3] Vascular claudication and overall deconditioning should be ruled out based on history and physical examination.[3]

Steppage gait patterns occur due to disturbance of lower motor neurons (LMNs).[2,5] Causes include peripheral neuropathy, lumbar radiculopathy, or sciatic neuropathy.[2] Foot drop results from weak ankle dorsiflexion and patients compensate by lifting the foot as high as possible, resulting in a gait with a waddling quality.[2,5] Ankle dorsiflexion weakness can also be elicited by having the patient attempt to walk on his or her heels.[2,3]

A parkinsonian gait is hypokinetic, rigid, and shuffling with decreased stride length, reduced arm swing, and loss of heel strike.[3,5] Patients may exhibit a lack of spontaneous movements, a flexed posture, and commonly a resting tremor that improves with initiation of movement.[2,5] Patients have difficulty initiating ambulation and when they do so, the trunk flexes forward and the lower extremities remain flexed.[2] Decreased step length results in a shuffling quality and festination later in the course of the disease.[2] Patients may also freeze when passing through a doorway, and turn en bloc.[2] A parkinsonian gait may improve with external cues but worsen when the patient is asked to perform a secondary task.[5,6] Drug-induced parkinsonism may occur secondary to neuroleptic drugs or Parkinson's-like condition such as PSP.

Ataxic gaits can occur due to cerebellar or sensory ataxia.[3] This gait pattern has an overall staggering, clumsy appearance necessitating a wide base.[3,5] The frontal gait of PSP is similar in appearance, but characteristically "reckless" due to the patient's lack of insight into fall risk (whereas patients with ataxic gaits are apprehensive).[3]

Sensory ataxic gait most commonly occurs due to diabetic polyneuropathy, but other causes include vitamin B12 deficiency and tabes dorsalis.[2] Patients stand with a wide base and keep their eyes on the ground due to impaired proprioception.[2] Loss of proprioception decreases patient awareness of limb position and the patients lift their legs high in the air, often producing a "slap" on the ground that increases sensory feedback.[2] A positive Romberg's sign (loss of balance standing after eyes close) indicates sensory ataxia or vestibular disease (whereas imbalance in cerebellar disease is present with eyes open and closed).[3]

Psychogenic gait presents with variable, inconsistent, and nonstereo-typical gait patterns, sometimes described as a "walking on ice" pattern.[3] The patient's gait on exam may even vary from the "unobserved" gait pattern seen when the patient enters the office.[3] Gait should not improve with backwards ambulation.[3] Bilateral leg buckling may be present, but patients remarkably maintain their balance.[3] In psychogenic hemiparesis, patients may excessively drag the limb (versus a patient with spastic dystonic gait who circumducts to clear the limb).[3] Facial expression should also be noted, and is commonly described as "la belle indifférence" in patients with psychogenic gait disturbance.[5] Dual tasking can also be performed and may show that patients with anxiety-related or psychogenic gait disturbance will tend to walk better when they are distracted by a second task.[7]

IMAGING STUDIES

Additional diagnostic tests may be performed selectively based on the presumed diagnosis that has been formulated on the basis of history and physical examination evidence.[7] Plain radiographs are indicated for patients exhibiting a Trendelenburg, antalgic, knee hyperextension, or other gaits related to limited joint mobility.[2] In any of these cases, plain radiographs of the involved region should be taken.[2]

Typical radiographs used to evaluate for knee osteoarthritis include standing anteroposterior (AP) and 45-degree flexion weight-bearing pos-teroanterior (PA) radiographs.[8] Subtle loss of joint space may be seen on 45-degree radiographs that does not appear on traditional extension views.[8]

Other changes that may be seen include osteophyte formation along the periphery of the tibia, flattening of the femoral condyles, and joint-space narrowing.[8] Weight-bearing AP radiographs including both extremities from the hips to the ankles may be useful in revealing angular deformity and allow determination of mechanical and anatomic axes of the limb.[8] If joint-space narrowing is present, magnetic resonance imaging (MRI) is not indicated, however, MRI may be performed in patients with minimal radiographic changes, localized pain, and clinical findings consistent with a meniscal abnormality.[8]

Imaging in the case of hip pathology should also start with plain radiographs to evaluate for osseous abnormalities or underlying arthropathy.[9] Standard hip radiographs include an AP view of the pelvis (allowing for visualization of both hips) as well as coned-down and "frog-lateral" views of the affected hip.[9] A groin lateral view of the hip keeps the hip in neutral position and may be used instead of the "frog-lateral" view in case of an acute femoral neck fracture.[9] Oblique or Judet views of the pelvis may be used in the case of a suspected acetabular fracture.[9] Since development of computed tomography (CT), plain radiographs of the hip are used less frequently (except to follow improvement in proximal femur fractures following treatment with open reduction and internal fixation, especially since plain radiographs are less degraded by metal artifact than CT).[9] Possible pathology seen on hip radiographs include joint space narrowing, fractures, erosions, osteophytes, osseous lesions, and soft tissue calcification or ossification.[9]

Conventional radiographs for the evaluation of disorders which localize to the spine may include AP and lateral views of the region of suspected pathology. Global spinal alignment can be assessed with standing full length PA and lateral radiographs to visualize the entire spine down to the bilateral femoral heads[6] (Figs. 10.3A and B). PA radiographs assess for coronal alignment and pelvic obliquity.[6] Lateral full-length radiographs provide assessment of sagittal and pelvic tilt.[6] Dynamic lateral views may also be indicated to evaluate for instability.[6] Plain radiographs may be supplemented by MRI to evaluate for evidence of neural compression and the integrity of neural elements.[2]

For a patient with a lesion which localizes to the brain, a CT is often the first study obtained. This imaging modality will identify evidence of hydrocephalus, intracranial hemorrhage, infarct, or mass effect. Further workup with MRI may be necessary to better delineate the etiology of the abnormality discovered on CT.

FURTHER WORKUP

In addition to qualitative observation, a quantitative gait analysis is useful to aid in the classification of gait disturbances.[7] Pressure-sensitive floors or

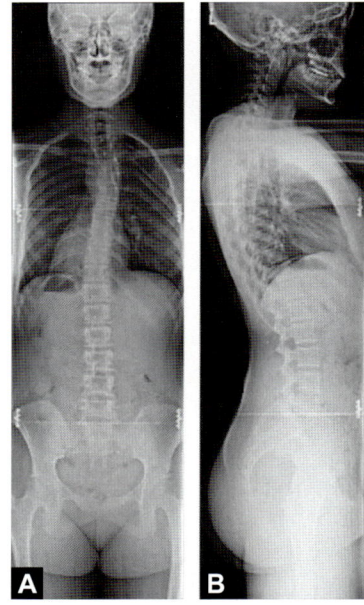

Figs. 10.3A and B: Posteroanterior (A) and lateral (B) full length standing radiographs.

three-dimensional registration of joint movements may be used to assess gait in a quantitative manner. Longitudinal assessment of patient progress can be quantitatively tracked via these methods.

In addition to radiographic studies, laboratory tests may aid in obtaining a diagnosis for the etiology of a gait disorder. Neuropathy most commonly occurs secondary to diabetes and a HbA1c level may be helpful in diagnosis.[2] Other causes of neuropathy may be investigated by testing for serum vitamin B12 and folate levels, serum rapid plasma reagin (RPR), and HIV screening.[2] Discontinuation of neurotoxic medications, including phenytoin, cisplatin and isoniazid may be diagnostic and therapeutic.[2]

Other useful tests for the evaluation of neuromuscular disorders are nerve conduction studies (NCS) and electromyography (EMG), creatinine kinase (CK) levels, repetitive nerve stimulation tests, and antibody studies.[4] Nerve conduction studies and EMG help localize the pathology and guide further diagnostic studies. Creatinine kinase level may be elevated in myopathic disorders, but also can be normal later in disease due to muscle atrophy.

REFERENCES

1. Sweeting K, Mock M. Gait and posture — assessment in general practice. Aust Fam Physician. 2007;36(6):398-401, 404-5.
2. Lim MR, Huang RC, Wu A, et al. Evaluation of the elderly patient with an abnormal gait. J Am Acad Orthop Surg. 2007;15(2):107-17.

3. Van Gerpen JA. Office assessment of gait and station. Semin Neurol. 2011; 31(1):78-84.

4. McDonald CM. Clinical approach to the diagnostic evaluation of hereditary and acquired neuromuscular diseases. Phys Med Rehabil Clin N Am. 2012; 23(3):495-563.

5. Snijders AH, van de Warrenburg BP, Giladi N, et al. Neurological gait disorders in elderly people: clinical approach and classification. Lancet Neurol. 2007;6(1):63-74.

6. Smith JS, Shaffrey CI, Fu KM, et al. Clinical and radiographic evaluation of the adult spinal deformity patient. Neurosurg Clin N Am. 2013;24(2):143-56.

7. Jahn K, Zwergal A, Schniepp R. Gait disturbances in old age: classification, diagnosis, and treatment from a neurological perspective. Dtsch Arztebl Int. 2010;107(17):306-15; quiz 316.

8. Cole BJ, Harner CD. Degenerative arthritis of the knee in active patients: evaluation and management. J Am Acad Orthop Surg. 1999;7(6):389-402.

9. Erb RE. Current concepts in imaging the adult hip. Clin Sports Med. 2001; 20(4):661-96.

CHAPTER 11

Sacroiliac Joint Pain

Martin Griffis, Jessica Stark, Daniel H Kim

INTRODUCTION

Chronic back pain is a common disorder with many different etiologies. Structures that have the potential to result in low back and lower extremity pain include herniated disk, nerve roots, spinal cord, ligaments, muscles, vertebrae and the sacroiliac joint (SIJ).[1] The SIJ is an often-overlooked cause of buttock and low back pain. In two large retrospective reviews looking at outpatients presenting for low back pain it was found that the SIJ was the genesis of 14–22% of low back pain.[2] Often, SIJ pain results from movements that place extra strain on the joint, its supporting ligaments, and its surrounding soft tissues.[3] Pain at the joint can be separated into two types: intra-articular (infection, arthritis, malignancies and spondyloarthropathies) and extra-articular (fractures, ligamentous injuries, leg length discrepancy, and myofascia).[4]

Arthritis is one of the most common causes of SIJ pain, with osteoarthritis being the most common form occurring at the SIJ; however, rheumatoid arthritis and post-traumatic arthritis are also common.[5] Pain generated in the SIJ can present as sacral pain, low back pain, pelvic pain, but is mainly localized in the gluteal region.[5] Most patients who present with SIJ pain secondary to arthritis describe a pain that is localized around the SIJ and upper posterior thigh, which radiates into the posterior buttocks (Fig. 11.1).[5] Pain typically does not radiate below the knee and is usually below the beltline, most often occurring unilaterally rather than bilaterally.[5] Pain is described as constant and achy, which usually worsens with an increase in physical activity.[5] Rest and heat have been shown to mitigate pain.[5]

It has been estimated that about 44–58% of patients who suffer from SIJ pain have a history of trauma.[5] SIJ pain is common in athletes, specifically in sports that require unilateral loading.[5] SIJ pain is more common in pregnant women, possibly due to the effect of the hormone relaxin, which increases joint laxity and range of motion.[3] Other contributing factors to SIJ pain include altered posture, scoliosis, leg length discrepancy, weight gain, and previous spinal fusions.[3,6]

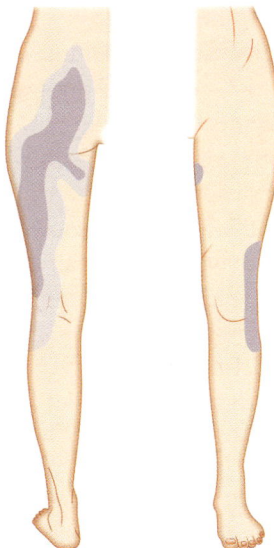

Fig. 11.1: Diagram showing common pain distribution seen in patients with sacroiliac joint pain. Pain generally is localized above the knee and below the beltline. *Source*: From Benzon HT, Rathmell JP, Wu CL, et al. Sacroiliac joint syndrome. Practical Management of Pain, 5th edition. Philadelphia, PA: Elsevier Mosby; 2014. pp. 866-75.[7]

DIFFERENTIAL DIAGNOSIS

- Arthritis including ankylosing spondylitis (AS)
- Sacroiliac joint dysfunction (microinstability)
- Lumbar radiculopathy
- Tumor
- Stress fracture
- Facet syndrome
- Degenerative disk disease
- Abdominal aortic aneurysm
- Nephrolithiasis
- Diverticular disease
- Referred pain from pelvic organs
- Herpes zoster
- Joint sepsis

Source: List taken from Miller MD, Hart JA, MacKnight JM. Sacroiliac joint. In: Miller MD (Ed.) Essential Orthopaedics. Philadelphia, PA: Saunders Elsevier; 2010. pp. 522-4.

ANATOMY

The SIJ, a diarthrodial synovial joint, is the largest axial joint in the body, connecting the sacrum with the bilateral pelvic bones (ilium).[6] Interestingly, only the anterior one third of the joint between the sacrum and the ilium is a true synovial joint.[6] The remaining portion of the joint is ligamentous.[6,8] The SIJ differs from others in that it has fibrocartilage in addition to hyaline cartilage, there is discontinuity of the posterior capsule, and the articular surface has many ridges and depressions. Multiple ligaments, fascia, and muscles attach across the joint, which limit its range of motion and provides stability.[9] The SIJ is stabilized by three core ligaments, which include the anterior sacroiliac ligament (ASL), posterior sacroiliac ligament (PSL) and interosseous ligaments.[9] In addition, three accessory ligaments, the sacrospinous ligament, sacrotuberous ligament and the iliolumbar ligament, provide further stabilization of the joint.[9]

Ventrally, the iliolumbar ligament strengthens the SIJ's superior margin.[9] The ASL stabilizes the anterior aspect of the SIJ capsule, while the superior portion of the sacrospinous ligament stabilizes the inferior aspect of the joint.[9] Dorsally, the SIJ is stabilized by the PSL, which is subdivided into short and long ligaments.[9] Within the SIJ is the interosseous sacroiliac ligament (ISL), which is the strongest of the SIJ supporting ligaments.[9] This ligament is responsible for providing multidirectional stability to the joint.[9]

Unlike most joints, no muscles act directly on the SIJ, however the network of muscles that are associated with the joint play a role in providing stability to the joint. The functional associations of the gluteus maximus, piriformis, and biceps femoris with the ligaments that stabilize the SIJ, provide further stability and indirectly influence joint mobility.[6] Motion at the SIJ is triplanar, occurring in all three planes, however mobility of the joint is not extensive, limited to about 2–4 degrees of rotation.[10]

A number of factors, including age and pregnancy can affect the SIJ.[6] The anterior surface (auricular surface) of the ilium, starting around puberty and continuing throughout life, is known to become rougher with age.[6] Around the 3rd or 4th decade of life, the most prominent changes in the SIJ occur, which include abnormalities with the joints surface and the aggregation of chondrocytes within the bone.[6] Age-related changes also occur within the sacrum, however they tend to come later in life, usually 10–20 years following the degenerative changes seen in the ilium.[6] During pregnancy, which is associated with increased weight gain and lordotic posture, the hormones relaxin and estrogen have been shown to increase joint ligamentous laxity which places women at a greater risk of experiencing SIJ pain.[6]

Innervation of the SIJ is quite controversial, and its exact innervation is unclear.[6,9] Generally, innervation at the SIJ is broken down into the innervation of the anterior aspect of the joint and that of the posterior aspect of the joint.[6,9] At the posterior aspect of the joint, innervation is thought to include the dorsal rami of spinal nerves L4-S3, however spinal nerves L3-S4 have been cited as well.[6,9] Innervation of the anterior aspect of the joint is the subject of much debate, however recent literature cites it as the anterior rami of spinal nerves L2-S2.[6]

Histologic analysis of the SIJ shows the presence of nerve fibers in the joint capsule and adjacent ligaments.[11] The capsular ligamentous tissue from the ventral aspect of the SIJ reveals both unmyelinated and myelinated nerve fascicles, individual axons, paciniform encapsulated mechanoreceptors and nonpaciniform mechanoreceptors.[11] This suggests that the joint itself can transmit pain and proprioception.

PHYSICAL EXAM

To diagnose SIJ pain, a multitude of SIJ provocative pain tests are currently used.[4,5] Typically, more than one provocative test is carried out in order to diagnose SIJ pain. Solitary provocative tests have been shown to have little diagnostic value, due to the high rate of false-positives.[4,5] On the contrary, multiple provocative tests can provide more discriminative power for diagnosing SIJ pain.[4] A recent study has shown that using 3 or more positive provocative tests resulted in a specificity and sensitivity ranging from 78–88% and 82–91%, respectively.[4,12] With this said, the value of multiple provocative tests is the subject of much debate; some authors citing its value, while a majority of studies demonstrating poor inter-examiner reliability.[6] Of the provocative tests used, six often used are listed below.

1. *Compression test (approximation test)*: This applies lateral compression force. The patient lies on their side with the affected side up; hips should be flexed to 45°, with the knees flexed to 90°. The examiner then applies a downward medial pressure on the anterior aspect of the lateral ilium between the greater trochanter and iliac crest in the direction of the contralateral ilium. Pain felt across the SIJ results in a positive test.[5]

2. *Patrick's sign (FABER test—flexion, abduction, and external rotation test)*: This applies tensile force. The patient lies supine with the examiner on the affected side. The patient places their foot on their affected side to the opposite knee. The patient's pelvis is stabilized at the opposite anterior superior iliac spine (ASIS) by the examiner's hand. Downward pressure is then applied to the knee on the affected side, guiding it toward the examining table. Pain elicited at the SIJ results in a positive test.[4,5,10]

3. *Distraction test (gapping test)*: This applies tensile forces on the anterior aspect of the SIJ. The patient lies supine with their forearm under the lumbar spine and the examiner on the patient's affected side. The examiner then places their hands on their ipsilateral ASIS and pressure is applied in a posterolateral direction. Asymmetrical movement or pain felt across the SIJ results in a positive test.[4]

4. *Gaenslen test (pelvic torsion test)*: The patient lies supine with their affected side on the edge of the examination table. The opposite hip and knee are maximally flexed toward their trunk, with the affected leg extended. Force is then applied to both the extended leg and the flexed knee. Pain felt at the SIJ is considered a positive test.[5,10]

5. *Gillet test (one-legged stork test)*: Patient is standing with the examiner positioned behind the patient. The examiner thumbs are placed on the patient's posterior superior iliac spine (PSIS) and the sacrum at the S2 level. The symptomatic hip is then flexed to 90°. A positive test results if the examiner's thumb is moved upward rather than inferomedially on the hip being flexed.[5] In a normal pelvis, the palpated side should move inferiorly with hip flexion, and a positive test indicates limited mobility.

6. *Sacral/thigh thrust test (posterior shear test)*: The patient lies supine with the unaffected leg extended and the examiner stabilizes the pelvis with a hand on the opposite ASIS. With the examiner on the affected side, the patient's hip is flexed to 90° with the knee bent. Axial pressure is placed along the length of the femur to draw the ilium posteriorly. Pelvic girdle pain results in a positive test.[5]

IMAGING STUDIES: MRI AND CT IMAGES

A challenging aspect of SIJ treatment is the difficulty of its diagnosis.[6] As mentioned previously, a number of pain provocation tests are available. Despite this abundance, studies have shown that these tests are often not consistent at accurately diagnosing SIJ pain.[6] Other than ruling out other sources of pain, imaging of the SIJ is not particularly useful in determining diagnosis.[3]

The SIJ's high susceptibility to stress fractures and tumors often warrants imaging which includes plain film radiography, computed tomography (CT), magnetic resonance imaging (MRI), and Doppler ultrasound of the lower lumbar spine and sacrum to help elucidate the source of the pain.[6] Radionuclide bone scanning is also occasionally used as a screening test for SIJ pain.[6] Similar to studies on pain provocative tests, studies examining radiography as a diagnostic aid show mixed results, with the majority showing little validity.[6] Currently, making a diagnosis and finding a treatment for SIJ pain is difficult since there is no specific gold standard imaging tests for diagnosis of SIJ pain.[10] Imaging of the joint is difficult due to the fact of multiple overlying soft tissue structures and the joint's location.[10]

When using plain film radiography to image the SIJ, the anteroposterior (AP) view should be taken aiming approximately 25°–30° cephalad. Lateral views are useful for diagnosing joint degeneration, tumors, demineralization and fractures.[10] CT scans are best at identifying osteoid osteomas, fractures and degeneration at the joint.[10] MRI is indicated when looking to identify tumors, soft-tissue pathology, fractures, lumbar disk disease and inflammatory diseases including sacroiliitis.[10] Lastly, Doppler ultrasound is best used to observe SIJ motion in patients who are pregnant.[10]

FURTHER WORKUP

Depending on clinical judgment and the patients' clinical presentation, additional testing such as complete blood count, erythrocyte sedimentation rate, human leukocyte antigen B27 (HLA-B27) genetic screening, and antinuclear antibody testing can be done.[5]

Patients with spondyloarthropathies, a broad category of inflammatory diseases, which affect bone, joints, ligaments and tendons, often complain of SIJ pain in the morning which improves with increasing activity.[13] Laboratory tests for these patients show markers of a nonspecific systemic inflammatory response.[13] For patients with AS, or suspected of having AS, screening for the HLA-B27 gene is often warranted.[13]

For diagnosing pain stemming from the SIJ, intra-articular fluoroscopically guided injections are often considered the closest diagnostic test to a gold standard.[3] For this test, the patient is prone and the joint is located using fluoroscopy.[3] Once the SIJ is identified, a needle is injected into the joint space by piercing the PSL (Figs. 11.2A to D).[3] A mixture of corticosteroid and local anesthetic is released into the joint space, blocking sodium ion channels of the nerves that innervate the SIJ.[3] This test can be diagnostic as well as therapeutic, as the corticosteroid may provide long-lasting relief.

TREATMENT

Treatment of SIJ pain can be divided into two major categories, treating the underlying cause and therapies aimed at alleviating symptoms.[6] Physical therapy, SIJ steroid injections under fluoroscopy, radiofrequency ablation, orthotics such as pelvic belts, prolotherapy (injecting chemical irritants into SIJ resulting in scarring of the joint), and SIJ fusion with instrumentation are the most common treatments. For spondylopathies, treatment typically includes medications such as antibiotics, nonsteroidal anti-inflammatory drugs (NSAIDs), oral steroids, methotrexate, cyclosporine, and bromocriptine.[6] Ligamentous and muscular pain can be relieved with anti-inflammatories and muscle relaxers as well as orthotics.

DISCUSSION

The SIJ is a complex joint that is an integral component of the axial support system. Given the inter-relationships of the SIJ with the spine, low back pain is commonly due to SIJ dysfunction. A thorough physical exam and imaging can rule out other causes of low back pain, increasing the likelihood of SIJ involvement. Conservative management with intra-articular injections and treatment of the underlying causes may provide relief, with SIJ fusion being

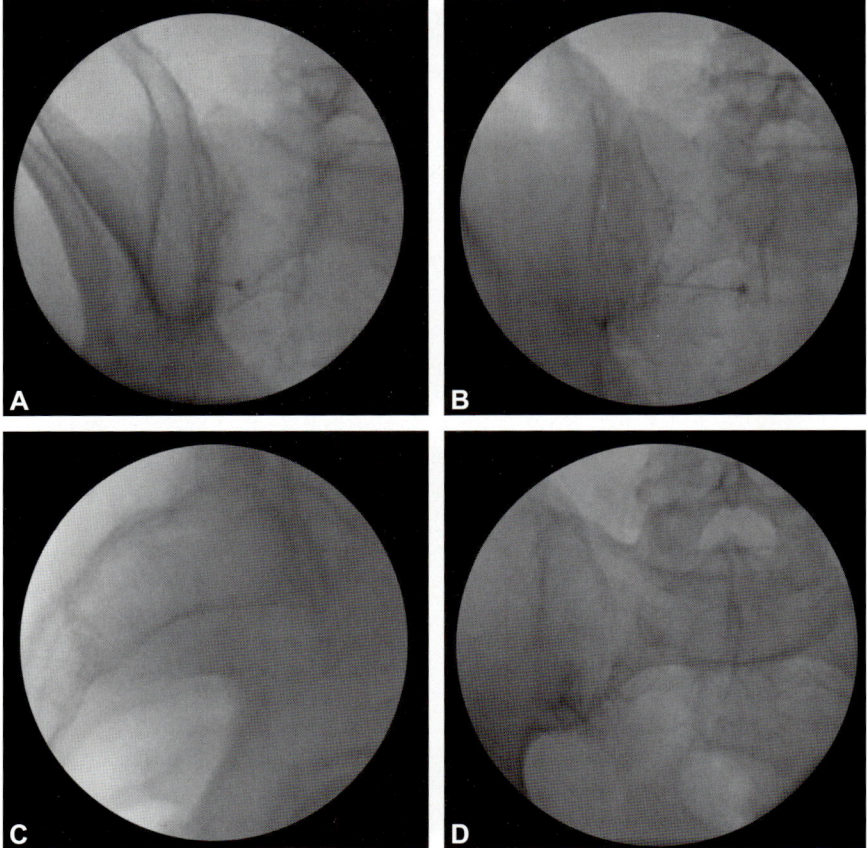

Figs. 11.2A to D: Figures show sacroiliac joint injection guided with fluoroscopy. *Courtesy*: Mitchell K. Freedman, DO.

a potential treatment for refractory cases. When evaluating patients with low back pain, the SIJ should always be considered as a potential source causing the pain.

REFERENCES

1. Hansen HC, Helm S. Sacroiliac joint pain and dysfunction. Pain Physician. 2003;6:179-89.
2. Cher D, Polly D, Berven S. Sacroiliac joint pain: burden of disease. Med Devices (Auckl). 2014;7:73-81.
3. Foley BS, Buschbacher RM. Sacroiliac joint pain: anatomy, biomechanics, diagnosis, and treatment. Am J Phys Med Rehabil. 2006;85(12):997-1006.
4. Vanelderen P, Szadek K, Cohen SP, et al. Sacroiliac joint pain. Pain Prac, 2010;10(5):470-8.
5. Waldman SD. Sacroiliac joint pain. Atlas of Common Pain Syndromes, 3rd edition. Philadelphia, PA: Saunders; 2012. pp. 256-9.

6. Cohen SP. Sacroiliac joint pain: a comprehensive review of anatomy, diagnosis and treatment. Anes Analg. 2005;101(5):1440-53.

7. Benzon HT, Rathmell JP, Wu CL, et al. Sacroiliac joint syndrome. Practical Management of Pain, 5th edition. Philadelphia, PA: Elsevier Mosby; 2014. pp. 866-75.

8. Benzon HT, Rathmell JP, Wu CL, et al. Radiologic assessment of the patient with spine pain. Practical Management of Pain, 5th edition. Philadelphia, PA: Elsevier Mosby; 2014. pp. 185-242.

9. Vleeming A, Schuenke MD, Masi AT, et al. The sacroiliac joint: an overview of its anatomy, function and potential clinical implications. J Anat. 2012;221(6): 537-67.

10. Miller MD, Hart JA, MacKnight JM. Sacroiliac joint. In: Miller MD (Ed.) Essential Orthopaedics. Philadelphia, PA: Saunders Elsevier; 2010. pp. 522-4.

11. Forst SL, Wheeler MT, Fortin JD, et al. The sacroiliac joint: anatomy, physiology, and clinical significance. Pain Physician. 2006;9(1):61-7.

12. Laslett M. Evidence-based diagnosis and treatment of the painful sacroiliac joint. J Man Manip Ther. 2008;16(3):142-52.

13. Asghar FA, Graziano GP, Kuntz C. Spondyloarthropathies (including ankylosing spondylitis). In: Winn RH (Ed). Youmans Neurological Surgery, 6th edition. Philadelphia, PA: Saunders Elsevier; 2011.

CHAPTER 12

Differential Diagnosis: Hemiparesis

Ahmed J Awad, Matthew Goldfarb, George M Ghobrial,
Christopher M Maulucci, James S Harrop

CHIEF COMPLAINT/HISTORY

Hemiparesis is defined as weakness on one side of the body with both the arm and leg involved. The word "hemi" means one side, while "paresis" means weakness. Hemiparesis should not be confused with hemiplegia which refers to the absence of motor strength (i.e. paralysis to both the upper and lower extremity on one side of the body).

Hemiparesis affects approximately 80% of patients with an intracerebral stroke, and as a result a high index of suspicion should be raised for an intracranial pathology. Patients that present to a spine clinic with the development of unilateral symptomatology of both the upper and lower extremities in tandem or in succession should undergo cranial imaging. Lesions causing hemiparesis will often result in upper motor neuron findings when intracranial and as a mixed upper and lower motor neuron lesion when affecting the cervical spinal cord. Lesions below the level of T1 spinal level typically will not cause upper extremity findings and hence hemiparesis can be localized to the brain and cervical spine (Box 12.1).

Patients usually present with a spastic or floppy arm, and with difficulty ambulating with a classic "circumduction gait" as shown in Figure 12.1.

Box 12.1: Common conditions presenting with hemiparesis.
• Stroke
• Cerebral palsy
• Traumatic brain injury
• Multiple sclerosis
• Congenital disorders of cerebral migration/development
• Brain tumors (primary or metastatic)
• Infections of the central nervous system
• Acute infantile hemiplegia

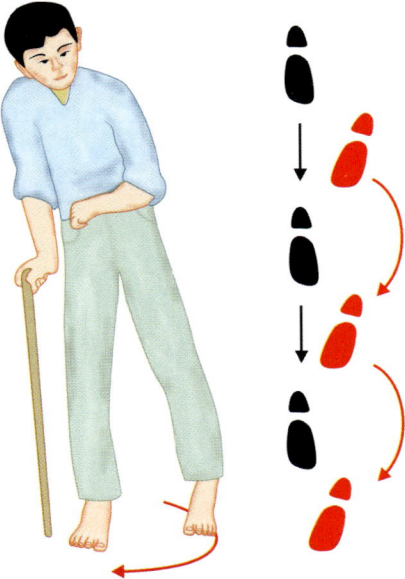

Fig. 12.1: The circumduction gait: A hemiparetic patient with a spastic paretic leg predominant with extensor tone.

This is characterized by unilateral loss of balance and precision in concert with muscle fatigue on the affected side of the body. Hemiparetic patients often have difficulties in performing daily life activities such as dressing, eating, using the bathroom and grabbing objects. These are the common findings that contribute to a decreased quality of life, although additional symptoms usually accompany weakness as will be discussed below.

DIFFERENTIAL DIAGNOSIS

The differential diagnosis of hemiparesis is numerous, and encompasses an expansive range of neuropathology (Box 12.1). However, with a thorough workup including a detailed history and physical, the spine clinician will be able to exclude several possible diagnoses. Moreover, establishing the time course of symptom onset is arguably one of the most important details to gather early in the patient encounter as this dictates the acuity of treatment as well as narrows the differential. A further discussion on the workup of hemiparesis will expand on this point.

WORKUP

The diagnosis of hemiparesis is based on examination while the underlying pathology can be narrowed down based on a careful medical history. A history of abrupt-onset of hemiparesis in a patient is a hallmark of a vascular event, most often an intracerebral stroke. This is the fourth-most common cause of death and a leading cause of permanent morbidity in adults. A history of a significant trauma should prompt cranial and spinal bony imaging followed by brain-specific imaging, with the intent on supporting a clinical diagnosis of traumatic brain injury.

As previously mentioned, a thorough understanding of neuroanatomy and good physical examination skills can effectively localize most lesions. Imaging studies then follow the neurologic examination for confirmation of the etiology and to determine the possible role for surgery. When a patient presents with hemiparesis, it is important to determine the pattern of muscle weakness. Most often, if a patient presents with hemiparesis from a spinal cord lesion there will be bilateral deficits with subtle findings on the contralateral side. Careful testing of all sensory modalities—pin prick, light and course touch, two-point discrimination, and proprioception is helpful as bilateral motor or sensory deficits is more common from a spinal cord lesion than a brain lesion.

Midline intracranial pathology such as a large, extra-axial, interhemi-spheric tumor (i.e. meningioma) could cause bilateral lower extremity weakness due to compression of the mesial primary motor fibers which supply the bilateral lower extremities. Intra-axial brain stem lesions that affect bilateral motor or sensory pathways are extremely rare, but can be ruled out with computed tomography (CT) and magnetic resonance imaging (MRI).

Types of Hemiparesis

- *Pure motor hemiparesis*: This is the most common one-sided hemiparesis. Patients experience unilateral weakness in their leg, arm and face. Facial motor involvement is a localizing sign of a cortical lesion.
- *Right-sided hemiparesis*: This is the result of pathology involving the left hemisphere, which results in language deficits in the majority of patients. Comprehensive testing of language includes comprehension, fluency, repetition, naming, and recall.
- *Cerebellum*: Damage to the cerebellum affects the ability of the body to coordinate movements, which can lead to problems with balance and posture known as, "ataxia". Pure cerebellar lesions should not result in hemiparesis, although ischemic lesions of the posterior circulation could affect corticospinal tracts and result in an ipsilateral hemiparesis if the lesion occurs below the pyramidal decussation, the point at which the motor fibers cross the midline.

IMAGING STUDIES

Improvements of radiographic techniques have enhanced the available tools that allow the clinician to make the proper diagnosis. The two most accurate imaging modalities are CT and MRI. CT is helpful in the early evaluation of osseous pathology, fractures, subluxation, acute hematoma, and acute ischemia.

Diffusion-weighted imaging (DWI) MRI is the most sensitive tool for stroke evaluation; however, the standard screening for stroke is a CT, not an MRI. This is due to the need for a rapid diagnosis of stroke and screening for potential intervention with a thrombolytic, followed by endovascular intervention upon meeting appropriate criteria.[7]

T1-weighted MRI with gadolinium is useful for evaluating for intra-axial neoplasms that may be missed on CT or non-contrasted T1 or T2 imaging. The presence of T1 or T2 signal changes or fluid attenuated inversion recovery (FLAIR) signal changes may aid in the diagnosis of an underlying pathologic process whose MRI changes are triggered by cytotoxic and/or vasogenic edema. T1-weighted imaging are necessary for the evaluation of high-grade neoplasms, demyelinating lesions, and infection, all of which can cause hemiparesis by direct extension into the motor fibers or by triggering inflammation in the adjacent somatosensory cortex.

FURTHER WORKUP

Further specialty techniques that may be useful are mainly noninvasive and invasive vascular imaging techniques for the purpose of working up stroke or transient ischemic attacks that manifest as hemiparesis. Magnetic resonance (MR) angiography is a noninvasive method of evaluating the great vessels of the neck, and the intracranial vasculature for stenosis, occlusion, atheromatous plaque, or aneurysm.

The addition of intravenous contrast to MR angiography can increase specificity greatly.[1-3,5] CT angiography is a time-delayed acquisition of high-resolution CT scans after intravenous contrast administration. This is considered the highest resolution noninvasive angiography available. The main drawback of this imaging technique is radiation exposure to the patient, but if performed properly, this risk is small compared to the potential for an accurate and proper diagnosis.[4] The risk of contrast nephropathy increases with the volume of contrast administered, and should be considered in the case of patients with pre-existing nephropathy. Pre-existing nephropathy is considered a potential contraindication for gadolinium administration due to the risk of nephrogenic systemic sclerosis (NSS), an extremely rare and sometimes fatal systemic reaction to gadolinium. The risk of NSS appears much lower than previously thought with the use of various gadolinium-based analogues.

Magnetic resonance imaging is helpful in spinal evaluation for underlying causes of hemiparesis. Intramedullary pathology includes syringomyelia, primary spinal cord tumors, spinal cord ischemia, and demyelinating lesions all of which could theoretically cause hemiparesis if affecting the cervical spinal cord. It is very rare that these disease processes would be manifest without any contralateral symptoms. Multiple sclerosis (MS) diagnosis can be made using a combination of MRI, neurologic findings, the clinical history, and the revised McDonald criteria issued by the National Multiple Sclerosis Society.[6]

There are a variety of laboratory techniques that can supplement the use of imaging to pinpoint a differential diagnosis.[8-9] The use of neurophysiology tools such as electromyography (EMG), and nerve conduction studies (NCS) can be especially helpful to diagnose neuromuscular diseases as well as distinguish upper and lower motor neuron lesions. EMG allows the physician to record and analyze the electrical activity produced by skeletal muscles. At rest, the normal muscle should be silent and no electrical signals should be detected. If abnormal electrical activity occurs during this silent state, such as fibrillation and fasciculations, this may indicate a primary nerve or muscle disorder. Fibrillation will occur about 2 weeks after the destruction or interruption of a motor neuron, and these denervated muscle fibers will begin to spontaneously activate. Fasciculations are involuntary contractions of the muscle, and may be either benign or indicative of an underlying neuromuscular disease. One should be aware of the amplitude and duration of the action potentials elicited from a muscle during EMG testing. Neuropathic diseases tend to have longer conduction time and higher relative amplitude than myopathic diseases.

Nerve conduction velocity is another useful laboratory technique to determine if problems exist with electrical conduction.[5] This technique works by stimulating motor nerves through the skin and then recording the action potentials in the muscle [compound muscle action potential (CMAP)]. One can then determine the distal latency, which is the time it takes for the impulse to travel from the site of conduction to the most distal electrode. Dividing the distance between these by the latency will provide a conduction velocity. Normal velocities range anywhere from 40–45 m/s to 70–75 m/s depending on the size and location of the muscle, as well as the age of the subject that is being studied. To find a conduction block one must stimulate the muscle at multiple sites, and can then infer that a demyelination of the nerve fiber exists.

CONCLUSION

Hemiparesis is a one side weakness that affects the majority of stroke patients. Hemiparesis can also be caused by brain tumors, MS and other diseases of the central nervous system. Patients usually present with a spastic or floppy arm, and circumduction gait. Pertinent medical history collection, thorough understanding of neuroanatomy and good physical examination skills can effectively localize the origin of muscle weakness. Imaging studies are helpful in confirming the clinical diagnosis. With the help of physical and occupational therapists, rehabilitation can help patients with hemiparesis to learn new ways of using their arms and legs and eventually regain movement and improve activities of daily living.

REFERENCES

1. Chimowitz, MI, Logigian, EL, Caplan, LR. The accuracy of bedside neurological diagnoses. Ann Neurol. 1990;28(1):78-85.
2. Bamford J, Sandercock P, Dennis M, et al. Classification and natural history of clinically identifiable subtypes of cerebral infarction. Lancet. 1991;337(8756): 1521-6.
3. Adams HP, Bendixen BH, Kappelle LJ, et al. Classification of subtype of acute ischemic stroke. Definitions for use in a multicenter clinical trial. TOAST. Trial of Org 10172 in Acute Stroke Treatment. Stroke. 1993;24(1):35-41.
4. Ropper AH, Samuels MA (Eds). Adams and Victor's Principles of Neurology, 10th edition. New York (NY): McGraw-Hill; 2014.
5. Filler AG, Kliot M, Howe FA, et al. Application of magnetic resonance in the evaluation of patients with peripheral nerve pathology. J Neurosurg. 1996; 85(2):299-309.
6. Polman CH, Reingold SC, Banwell B, et al. Diagnostic criteria for multiple sclerosis: 2010 revisions to the McDonald criteria. Ann Neurol. 2011;69(2):292-302.
7. Hagmann P, Jonasson L, Maeder P, et al. Understanding diffusion MR imaging techniques: from scalar diffusion-weighted imaging to diffusion tensor imaging and beyond. Radiographics. 2006;26 Suppl 1:205-23.
8. Latchaw RE (Ed). MRI and CT Imaging of the Head, Neck, and Spine, 2nd edition. St. Louis (MO): Mosby; 1991.
9. Van Doorn PA, Ruts L, Jacobs BC. Clinical features, pathogenesis, and treatment of Guillain-Barré syndrome. Lancet Neurol. 2008;7(10):939-50.

CHAPTER 13

Progressive Diffuse Paresis in Adults

Kevin Henrichsen, Sarah Nyirjesy, Saint-Aaron Morris

INTRODUCTION

Diffuse paresis can have a variety of clinical presentations, and may be a solitary finding or an element in a constellation of symptoms. The clinician must have a systematic approach to the patient as some entities may threaten life and/or function. This chapter will address the common disorders that can impact various levels of the neuromuscular axis in order to organize the examiner's thought process, and is organized in subsections that will examine cranial, spinal, peripheral nerve, neuromuscular junction, and muscular pathology. One of the most important elements in this approach is recognition of disease patterns in both the history and physical examination, which should prompt the clinician of the appropriate workup.

INTRACRANIAL DISORDERS

Intracranial disease processes are unified by their ability to alter consciousness, generate headaches and cervical pain, as well as cause a mixture of focal findings in conjunction with weakness. Similar to intrinsic spinal cord insults, longstanding intracranial pathology is associated with the development of upper motor neuron (UMN) findings when the corticospinal tracts are affected. This is characterized by the development of hypertonia and hyperreflexia in the setting of paresis or plegia (UMN signs). Patients will also develop upgoing plantar reflexes due to disinhibition of tonic cerebellospinal input. Maintaining a working knowledge of the motor pathways will further aid in localizing these lesions to the cerebrum, brain stem, and spinal cord (Fig. 13.1). Each segment of the brain stem contains unique cranial nerve functions that will further aid in localization. Midbrain lesions will have the capacity to affect oculomotor and trochlear nerve functions while pontine lesions will have the ability to affect trigeminal and abducens nerve relays. Finally, insults to the medulla may directly affect facial, vestibulocochlear, glossopharyngeal, vagus, hypoglossal, and spinal accessory nerve activity.

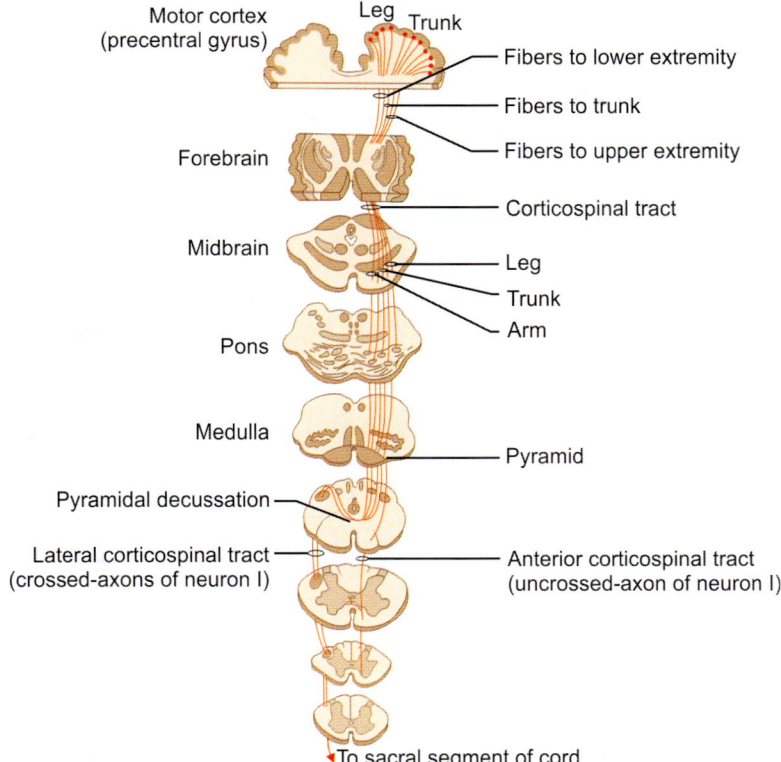

Fig. 13.1: Motor pathways of the CNS.

Chronic Subdural Hematoma

Chronic subdural hematomas are collections of old blood between the dura mater and brain parenchyma. Chronic subdural hematomas generally affect people between the ages of 50 years and 70 years and become noticeable weeks or months after minor trauma. Patients may present with unilateral paresis of the extremities, altered mentation, headaches, recurrent falls, and sometimes seizures.[1] Any patient with persistent altered mentation or focal deficit should undergo computed tomography (CT).[2] Imaging will typically reveal a mixed density to hypodense accumulation overlying a cerebral convexity (Fig. 13.2). However, magnetic resonance imaging (MRI) is indicated in those who have subtle lesions that may have gone unnoticed during initial CT screening.[1]

Intracranial Tumors

Intracranial tumors can be either primary or secondary, and metastases account for the overwhelming majority. In the adult population, brain tumors have a propensity to affect the supratentorial compartment.[3] Consequently,

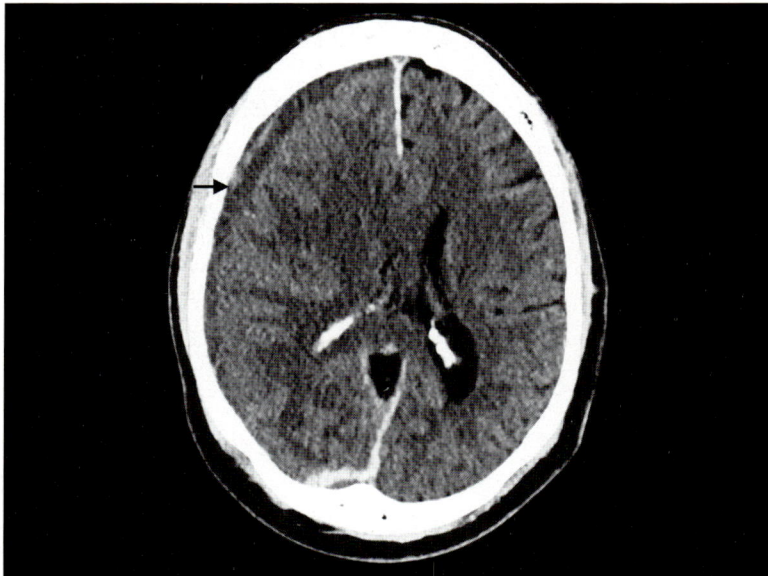

Fig. 13.2: CT head without contrast has arrow demonstrating hypodense right convexity subdural collection in a patient that presented with 2-week history of headaches and left hemiparesis.

patients with brain tumors may present with varying focal deficits. Common complaints are headaches that tend to be worse upon awakening due to increased intracranial pressure, altered mental status, nausea/vomiting, weakness, sensory abnormalities, and seizures. A head CT is indicated in this setting and MRI brain with and without contrast should be obtained once the suspicion of brain tumor has arisen.[4]

Moyamoya Disease

Moyamoya disease is a disease of the cerebrovasculature, specifically around the circle of Willis. It primarily affects Japanese patients but does affect all races.[5] Women are almost twice as likely to be diagnosed with Moyamoya as men and the highest incidences of the disease are found in patients in the 1st and 3rd–5th decades of life.[6] In adults, Moyamoya is most likely to present due to sudden rupture of a collateral vessel while children and adolescents are more likely to experience ischemic events.[6,7] Symptoms may vary depending upon the affected territory, and may include headaches, sensory dysfunction, involuntary movements, hemiparesis, and seizures.[6] Cerebral angiography is indicated for suspected Moyamoya although computed tomographic angiography (CTA) and magnetic resonance angiography (MRA) can be performed for screening.[7] The relevant imaging findings include: bilateral

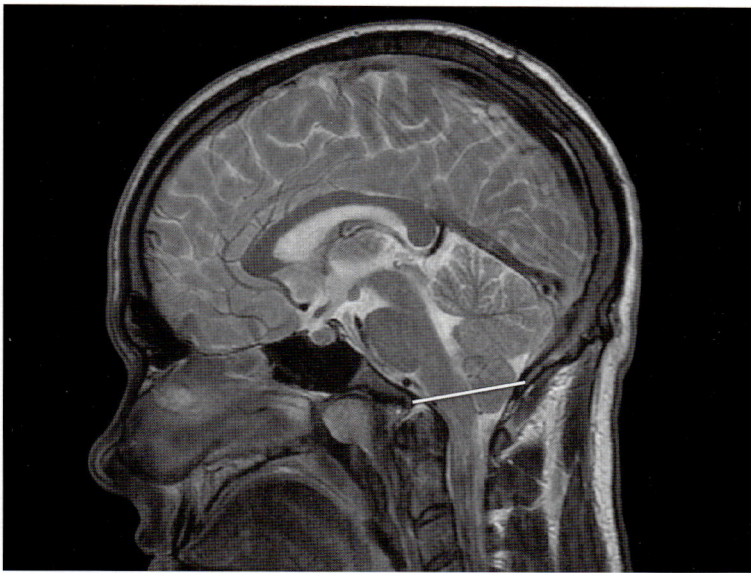

Fig. 13.3: T2-weighted sagittal MRI brain has line demonstrating cerebellar tonsils extending 5 mm beyond the foramen magnum in a patient complaining of headaches, cervicalgia, and difficulty using distal upper extremities.

occlusion or stenosis of the distal intracranial carotid artery or proximal anterior and middle cerebral arteries and atypical capillary networks near affected segments.[8]

Chiari Malformations

Chiari malformations represent abnormalities in hindbrain descent and cerebrospinal fluid (CSF) hydrodynamics that may cause myelopathy and hydrocephalus and/or syrinx formation, respectively. Chiari I and Chiari II are the most common subtypes, and are associated with varying degrees of cerebellar tonsil descent.[9] Chiari I tends to affect adults and older children with a slight female predominance while Chiari II is more common in infants and younger children.[10,11] Patients with Chiari I present with headaches and neck pain worsened by maneuvers that increase intracranial pressure (i.e. coughing, straining), as well as weakness and paresthesias from the presence of syringes.[12] Diagnosis can be made in a patient with an MRI of the brain and cervical spine that demonstrates at least 5 mm of cerebellar tonsil descent with or without the presence of a syrinx (Fig. 13.3).[13]

Multi-Infarct Dementia

Multi-infarct dementia (MID) is a loss of brain function caused by several small strokes. MID is most commonly diagnosed in people aged 55–75 years and is more prevalent in men than women. Patients with MID present with stepwise decline in memory and other cognitive functions, as well as other signs of stroke such as hemiparesis, sensory loss, aphasia, and UMN signs.[14-16] CT of the head will show signs of encephalomalacia while MRI of the brain will demonstrate restricted diffusion in various white matter regions.

Spinal Cord Disorders

Similar to intracranial disease processes, spinal cord dysfunction is characterized by the presence of UMN signs. Lower motor neuron (LMN) findings may also be present in the setting of demyelinating diseases that affect the anterior horn cells solely, as it houses the second-order cell bodies of the peripheral motor nerve processes. Concomitant sensory deficits are often present in patients with spinal cord disease and identifying a sensory level is a useful adjunct in determining which spinal regions necessitate imaging with CT or MRI. Furthermore, recognizing incomplete spinal cord presentations will aid the examiner in generating the most likely differential diagnoses when there is no clear source of spinal cord insult.

Transverse Myelitis

Transverse myelitis (TM) most commonly presents in either the 2nd or 4th decade of life. Many pediatric cases have a recent history of immunization or an illness that was followed by fever, nausea, and myalgia. It typically presents with progressively worsening weakness and sensory dysfunction.[17] The symptoms generally reach a nadir at least 4 hours following onset.[18] Adults more commonly present with paresthesias, sexual dysfunction, and bowel/bladder incontinence.[17] Magnetic resonance imaging of the suspected spinal levels should be performed, as well as lumbar puncture. magnetic resonance imaging will demonstrate a demyelinating plaque and T2 hyperintensity around active lesions. Cerebrospinal fluid and serum studies should be assessed for autoantibodies and infectious workup.[18]

Multiple Sclerosis

Multiple sclerosis (MS) is an autoimmune inflammatory disease that affects the axons of the central nervous system, demyelinating them and generally causing a variable course of multifocal deficits. Multiple sclerosis classically causes episodic neurologic deficits that resolve and have a stable symptom-free period (relapsing-remitting). However, in about 30% of cases there may be some degree of progression. Multiple sclerosis is almost 2.5 times more common in women than men and the typical age of onset is between the 2nd and 5th decades of life.[20] The disease has predilection for the brain, optic nerve, and spine. Presentation may include painful vision

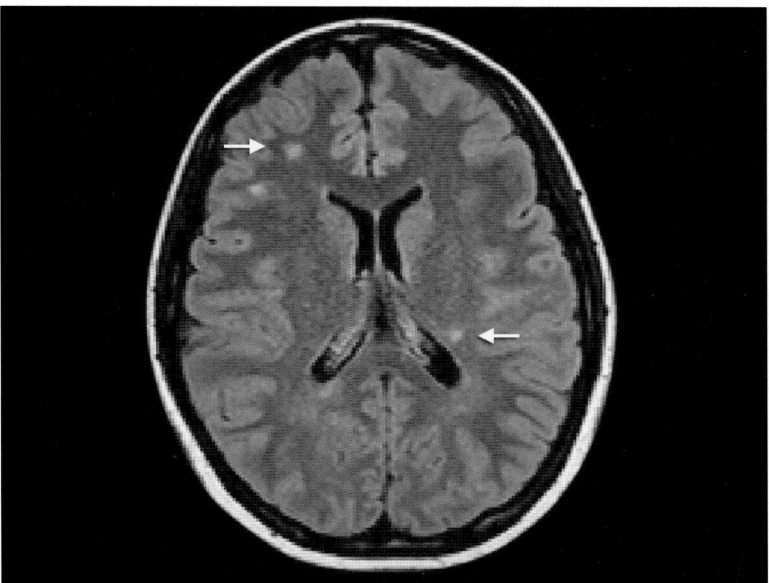

Fig. 13.4: T2 fluid-attenuated inversion recovery (FLAIR) axial MRI brain has arrows showing two periventricular demyelinating lesions in a patient experiencing a multiple sclerosis (MS) flare.

---

loss (optic neuritis), diplopia, hemi/monoparesis, paresthesias, sensory ataxia, autonomic dysfunction (bladder, bowel, or sexual dysfunction), and cognitive dysfunction.

Physical examination may reveal UMN findings, impaired proprioception from dorsal column involvement, diplopia, Lhermitte's sign (shock-like sensation down the back following neck flexion), and wide-based gait. Initial labs should be performed to rule out collagen vascular disease, infections such as Lyme disease and syphilis, endocrine abnormalities, sarcoidosis, vasculitides, or vitamin B_{12} deficiency. Magnetic resonance imaging brain and cervical spine are indicated for diagnosis and may demonstrate both active and healing plaques along the white matter tracts. Lesions of the brain are classically periventricular (Fig. 13.4).[19,21] Cerebrospinal fluid analysis should also be performed and assessed for both IgG levels and oligoclonal bands, which are sensitive but nonspecific indicators of disease.[22] *See* the McDonald criteria for clinical diagnosis (Table 13.1).[19]

Spinal Stenosis

The primary symptom of patients with any form of spinal stenosis is pain. When stenosis is severe enough, the spinal cord and/or nerve roots can become impinged and cause myelopathy or radiculopathy, respectively. Pain from spinal stenosis is estimated to affect approximately 75% of the general

Table 13.1: McDonald criteria for clinical diagnosis.

Clinical presentation (attacks)	Lesions	Additional data needed to make diagnosis
2	Objective evidence of ≥ 2 lesions or objective evidence of 1 lesion with history of prior attack	None
≥2	Objective evidence of 1 lesion	Dissemination in space, demonstrated by: • T2 lesion in at least two MS typical CNS regions (periventricular, juxtacortical, infratorial, spinal cord); *Or* • Await further clinical attack
1	Objective evidence of ≥2 lesions	Dissemination in time, demonstrated by: • Simultaneous asymptomatic contrast-enhancing and non-enhancing lesions at any time; *Or* • A new T2 and/or contrast-enhancing lesion(s) on follow-up MR irrespective of its timing; *Or* • Await a second clinical attack
1	Objective evidence of 1 lesion	Dissemination in space: • T2 lesion in at least two MS typical CNS regions; *Or* • Await further clinical attack *and* Dissemination in time, demonstrated by: • Simultaneous asymptomatic contrast-enhancing and non-enhancing lesions at any time; *Or* • A new T2 and/or contrast-enhancing lesions(s) on follow-up MR, irrespective of its timing; *Or* • Await a second clinical attack
0		1 year of disease progression (retrospective or prospective) *and* at least 2 out of 3 criteria: • Dissemination in space in the brain: one T2 lesion in periventricular, juxtacortical or infratentorial regions • Dissemination in space in the spinal cord: 2 T2 lesions; *Or* Positive CSF

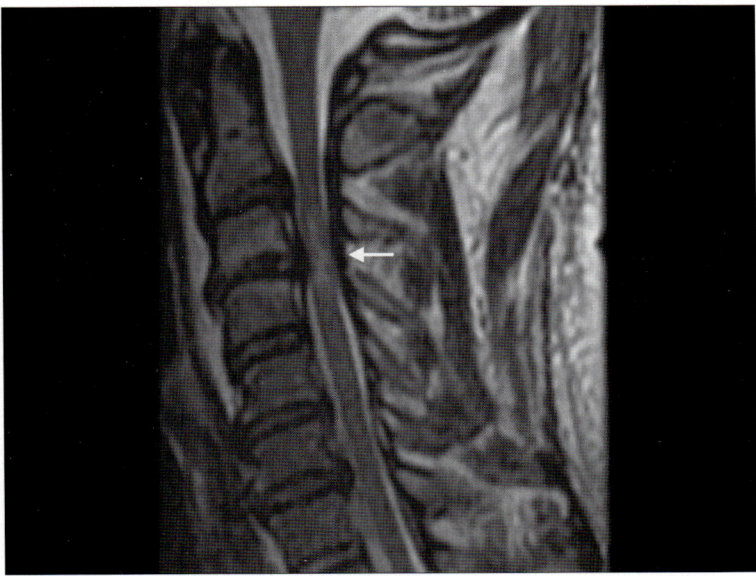

Fig. 13.5: T2-weighted sagittal MRI cervical spine has arrow showing cervical cord contusion from a large C3 disk herniation in a patient with worsening myelopathy.

population by the age of 60 years.[23,27] Cervical spinal stenosis may be defined as an anteroposterior (AP) spinal canal diameter less than 10 mm, and common offenders include ligamentum flavum hypertrophy, bony spondylitic changes, and facet hypertrophy. Consequently, patients may present with symptoms of loss of hand dexterity, difficulty with ambulation, paresthesias, and cervicalgia.[25] In more severe cases, there may be symptoms of urinary and fecal incontinence due to autonomic dysfunction.[25,28] Furthermore, the comprised spinal canal poses heightened risk for spinal cord injury in the setting of trauma and patients may become acutely quadriparetic/plegic. On examination, UMN signs may be present, which include a positive Hoffman's sign (flicking the nail bed of middle finger causes reflexive finger flexion). In addition, sensation may be diminished in accordance with the affected dermatomes.[28] Magnetic resonance imaging should be obtained of the cervical spine for further evaluation or CT myelogram of the cervical spine can be performed in those with contraindications to MRI (Fig. 13.5).[26]

Lumbar spinal stenosis (LSS) is typically associated with narrowing of the spinal canal to less than 12 mm in diameter. Similarly, patients present with lower back pain, muscle spasms, lower extremity weakness, or numbness of the legs that is worse when active and alleviated by rest (neurogenic claudication). Lumbar flexion, sitting down, or stationary biking tend to alleviate pain as this increases spinal canal and neural foramina diameter while extension decreases it during buckling of the ligamentum flavum and reapproximation of the facet joints.[27,30] Patients will have LMN findings

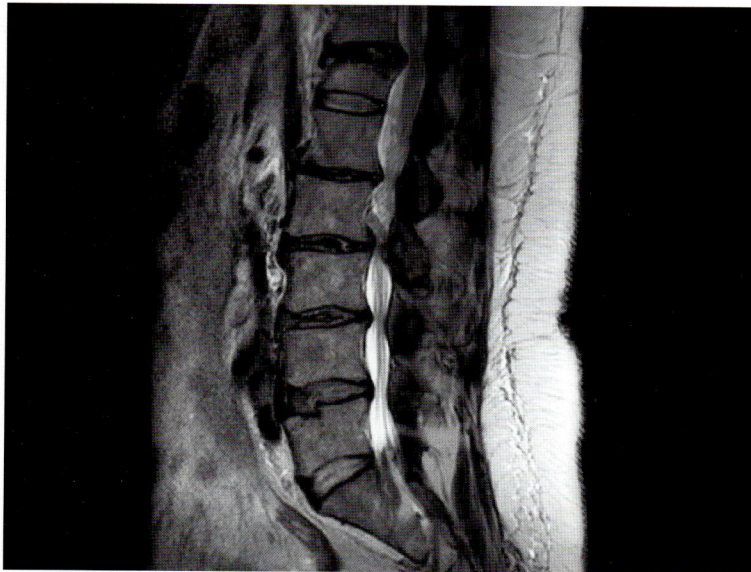

Fig. 13.6: T2-weighted sagittal MRI lumbar spine demonstrates severe multilevel lumbar stenosis that is worse at L1-2 and L2-3.

(decreased strength, hyporeflexia, and downgoing plantar reflexes) in most cases but the conus medullaris may be occasionally compromised and create UMN findings.[27] Magnetic resonance imaging lumbar spine (Figs. 13.6 and 13.7) is the modality of choice for assessment and CT lumbar myelograms can be used in those with contraindications to MRI.[24,29] In addition, nerve conduction studies (NCS) and electromyography (EMG) are useful adjuncts in discriminating LSS from other possible sources of neuropathy when imaging findings are unimpressive or perplexing.[31]

Spinal Epidural Abscess

Spinal epidural abscesses typically have an associated osteomyelitis, and generally occur in those greater than 50 years of age.[34] Common risk factors include immunosuppressive conditions [human immunodeficiency virus (HIV), chronic steroid use, chemotherapy treatment, and diabetes], alcoholism, renal failure, and intravenous (IV) drug abuse.[33,34] Patients generally complain of severe back pain that progresses if untreated to cause radiculopathy and myelopathy. Symptoms may also acutely worsen following a minor trauma in the setting of pathologic fractures from osteomyelitis. Physical examination will reveal tenderness to palpation along affected regions, there may be LMN or UMN findings, as well as sensory abnormalities.[33,34] Laboratory testing should include baseline C-reactive protein, erythrocyte sedimentation rate, complete blood count (CBC), and blood cultures.[32,33] Patients should undergo MRI with and without contrast of the affected spinal levels (Fig. 13.8).[33,34]

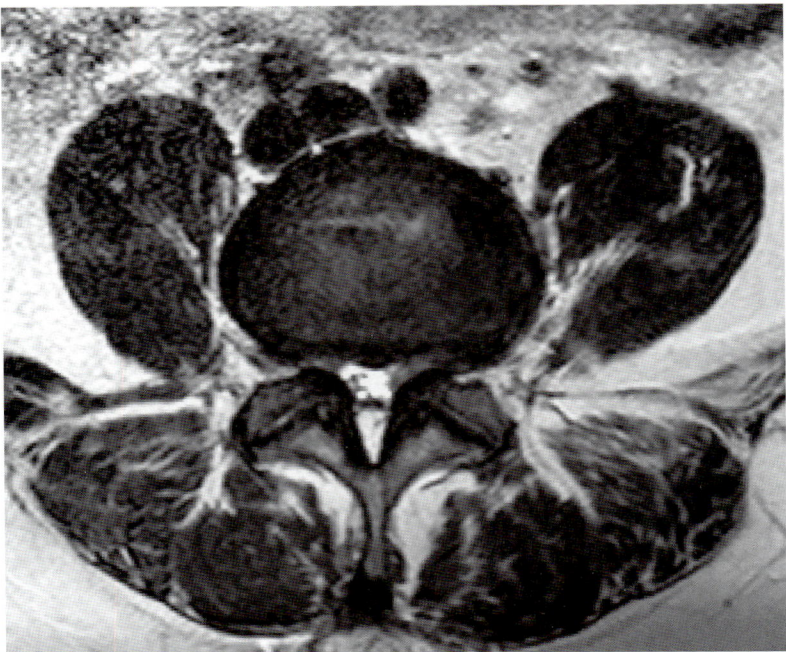

Fig. 13.7: T2-weighted axial MRI lumbar spine from same patient shows severe hypertrophy of the ligamentum flavum and facets.

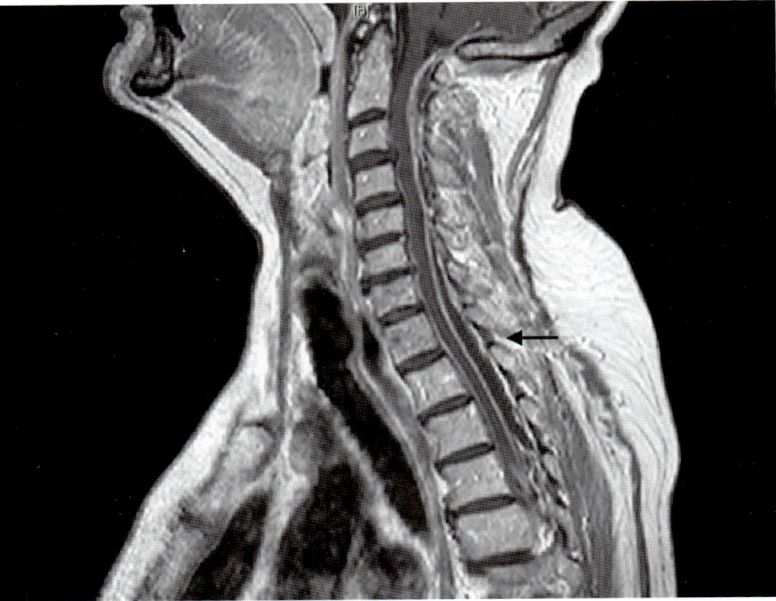

Fig. 13.8: T1-weighted sagittal MRI thoracic spine with contrast has arrow pointing to extensive dorsally-based spinal epidural abscess in a patient with worsening back pain, quadriparesis, and incontinence.

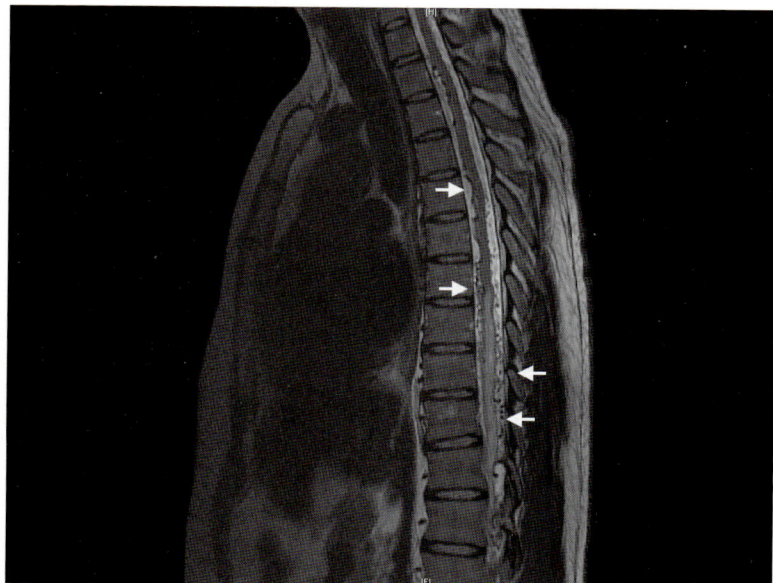

Fig. 13.9: T2-weighted sagittal MRI thoracic spine has various arrows highlighting serpiginous flow voids that are suggestive of an underlying spinal vascular malformation.

Spinal Vascular Malformations

The most common spinal vascular malformation (SVM) is the dural arteriovenous fistulas (AVFs). They are characterized by the abnormal communication of a radicular artery feeding directly into a spinal vein, usually in the thoracolumbar region.[35-37] This occurs most frequently in males over the age of 40. Type II and III intradural AVFs occur within the spinal parenchyma while type IV lesions may be found along the cord.[36,37] These entities represent direct communication between a spinal artery and a spinal vein and commonly occur in patients between 20 years and 50 years of age.[38]

In more than 80% of patients, symptoms are due to venous congestion from the high arterial flow. Consequently, patients may develop progressive myelopathy, radiculopathy, and back pain (Foix-Alajouanine syndrome). The remaining subset of patients may have sudden back pain and neurological deterioration due to hemorrhage. Patients may have varying degrees of UMN and LMN findings on examination, and localization may be impacted by the extent of venous congestion and subsequent neurologic dysfunction.[38,39] Magnetic resonance imaging of the spine should be performed and will demonstrate extramedullary flow voids (80%) and may also demonstrate T2 signal changes of the cord due to spinal cord edema and/or syrinx (Fig. 13.9).[40] Spinal angiography is necessary for complete evaluation and treatment planning (Fig. 13.10).[39,40]

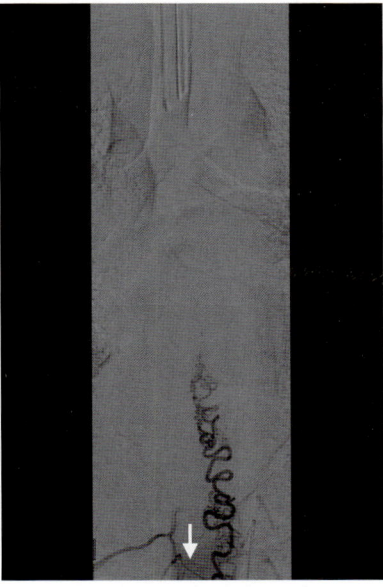

Fig. 13.10: Spinal thoracic angiogram performed on previous patient has arrow demonstrating fistula at level of radicular artery that is causing early filling of spinal veins.

Spinal Cord Tumors

The majority of spinal cord tumors are metastatic tumors and account for 85% of cases of neoplastic spinal cord compression. Metastatic spinal cord tumors are most common in individuals more than 50 years of age. It is estimated that 5–10% of patients with known cancer will develop spinal metastasis. The most common primaries to do so include: lung, breast, prostate, renal, lymphoma, and multiple myeloma.[41] Primary spinal cord tumors occur slightly more frequently in males and the majority of primary tumors occur in people between the 4th decade and 6th decade of life.[42]

The preponderance of intramedullary primary spinal cord tumors are glial tumors or ependymomas while extramedullary primary spine tumors are typically schwannomas, meningiomas, and neurofibromas. Spinal cord compression due to neoplasms may present with a constellation of findings such as worsening back pain, muscle stiffness, abnormal posture, weakness, sensory loss, paresthesias, or autonomic dysfunction depending upon disease extent.[43,44] Syndromes of incomplete spinal cord involvement may be present as well. For instance, the presence of a syrinx may cause a central cord presentation in those with cervical involvement. Lesions with a significant degree of laterality may also cause a hemicord syndrome. Finally, Lhermitte's sign may be present in those with a cervical mass due to heightened neuronal sensitivity.[43-45]

Magnetic resonance imaging of the suspected levels of disease should be performed with and without contrast. Metastatic bone disease preferentially affects the posterior vertebral bodies and typically extends posteriorly towards the canal. Additionally, pathological compression fractures may be present in this setting from compromise of the bony elements. Computed tomography imaging of the spine can also be utilized to assess bone integrity for operative planning.[44]

PERIPHERAL NERVE DISORDERS

Conditions affecting the peripheral nerve are a robust subject area; however, this section will focus on common sources associated with diffuse paresis from polyneuropathy. During the assessment of patients with diffuse paresis secondary to peripheral nerve dysfunction, the examiner will notice the affected limbs to be hypotonic, hyporeflexic, and with varying degrees of sensory dysfunction. Furthermore, as the disease progresses the affected muscles begin to lose bulk due to impaired transport of trophic factors. With this in mind, the patient may experience hypesthesia (diminished sensation), dysesthesia (pain during non-noxious stimulation), and paresthesias (numbness and tingling) in the respective dermatome. It is important that the examiner be familiar with the dermatomal distribution and muscle innervation of the various spinal nerves in order to distinguish nerve root lesions from more distal spinal nerve and peripheral nerve lesions (Fig. 13.11 and Table 13.1).

Amyotrophic Lateral Sclerosis

Amyotrophic lateral sclerosis (ALS) causes progressive motor neuron death, which leads to paralysis and eventual respiratory failure. The majority of ALS cases are sporadic, whereas 10% are inherited. The incidence is 1–2 per 100,000.[45] Typically ALS begins as slight weakness in the distal aspect of a single limb. The patient may notice difficulty performing fine motor tasks, atrophy of the muscles of one hand, or difficulty ambulating. Clinically both UMN and LMN signs are present. Cramping, stiffness, and fasciculations are also commonplace as the disease progresses to the remaining limbs while sparing sensation. ALS is a diagnosis of exclusion after all other potential causes of gradually worsening UMN and LMN signs have been ruled out.[46] EMG can reveal clinical and subclinical LMN involvement, as well as features of denervation and reinnervation. NCS are typically used to exclude other disorders.[46]

Guillain-Barré Syndrome

Guillain-Barré syndrome (GBS) is a common cause of acute paresis and paralysis. Population-based studies have found the incidence of GBS to be 0.6–4 cases per 100,000. Males have a 50% higher incidence than females. Incidence also tends to increase with age.[47] GBS is subdivided into several

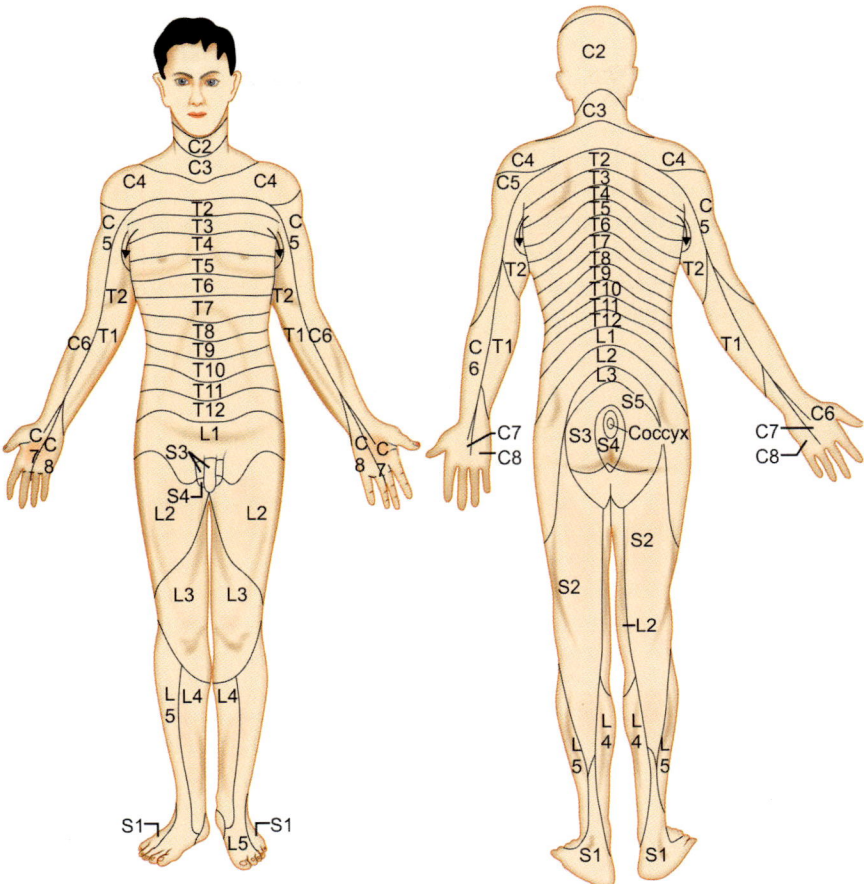

Fig. 13.11: Dermatomal distribution of the body.

subtypes, the most common are acute inflammatory demyelinating polyradi-culoneuropathy (AIDP), acute motor axonal neuropathy (AMAN), and acute motor and sensory axonal neuropathy (AMSAN). AIDP accounts for 90% of GBS cases in North America and Europe. In Asia and South America, 30–47% of cases are of the axonal subtypes. Two-thirds of cases are preceded by flu-like illness or gastroenteritis about 6 weeks prior to symptom onset. A variety of bacterial and viral causes have been identified with *Campylobacter jejuni* being the most common antecedent infection.[48] Rarely GBS has been seen following influenza vaccinations.

Acute inflammatory demyelinating polyradiculoneuropathy presents in a typical pattern: the patient will experience paresthesias in the digits of the hands and feet, and over a period of days to weeks there is symmetrical ascending weakness. The lower extremities are affected first followed by the upper extremities. Both proximal and distal muscle groups will be involved.

Weakness of the trunk, neck, and cranial muscles may occur later in the disease course. A minority of patients will experience total paralysis with respiratory failure. In addition to the paresis, patients may experience aching pain in the thighs and back, sensory dysfunction, and loss of deep tendon reflexes. The disease usually peaks at 2–4 weeks and recovery occurs over a period of weeks to months.

When the patient's presentation is concerning for GBS, CSF analysis is diagnostic. It will show an elevated protein concentration in 80% of cases and is either acellular or contains few lymphocytes (albuminocytologic dissociation).[1] NCS will frequently show a reduction in the compound muscle action potential (CMAP), partial motor conduction block, slowed conduction velocity, prolonged distal latencies, and reduced distal amplitudes. In a small percentage of cases the NCS will be normal, warranting repeat testing in 1–2 weeks.[47]

Porphyric Polyneuropathy

An exacerbation of acute intermittent porphyria can cause symptoms of severe motor polyneuropathy that resembles GBS. Although rare, this presents as symmetrical, progressive weakness of the extremities. Unique symptoms include colicky nausea and vomiting, abdominal pain, and constipation. Diagnosis is based on elevated levels of aminolevulinic acid and porphobilinogen in the urine during an acute attack. Unlike GBS, the CSF will appear normal and NCS will show diminished CMAPs in the absence of demyelination.[49]

Chronic Inflammatory Demyelinating Polyradiculoneuropathy

Chronic inflammatory demyelinating polyradiculoneuropathy (CIDP) is a slow and progressive disorder of peripheral nerves that leads to symmetric sensorimotor loss and areflexia of both proximal and distal muscle groups. The final presentation of this disorder is strikingly similar to GBS; however, CIDP slowly advances over a period of more than 2 months. Diagnosis is based both on clinical presentation and electrophysiological testing. Similar to GBS, NCS has findings consistent with demyelination. Cerebrospinal fluid analysis is also similar to GBS with respect to the presence of albuminocytologic dissociation.[50]

NEUROMUSCULAR JUNCTION DISORDERS

Neuromuscular junction disorders share similar characteristics. Fluctuation in the severity of the symptoms is the most striking commonality. Recognition of patterns in the characteristic fluctuating fatigue is crucial in the diagnosis of these disorders.

Myasthenia gravis (MG) is an autoimmune disorder caused by auto-antibodies against nicotinic acetylcholine receptor, muscle-specific kinase (MuSK), or lipoprotein-related protein 4 (LRP4). It is the most common cause of neuromuscular junction (NMJ) disorders and has an incidence between 1.7 cases per million and 21 cases per million and prevalence between 15 per million and 179 per million.[51] There is a bimodal distribution with higher prevalence in females in the 3rd–4th decade of life and equal distribution between sexes in the 7th–9th decade of life.[52] Myasthenia gravis will typically present as painless weakness of the ocular muscles causing ptosis and diplopia, but patients may also present with weakness of the bulbar muscles and/or proximal muscle groups of the limbs. Muscle weakness generally worsens later in the day and after prolonged use.

Lambert-Eaton myasthenic syndrome (LEMS) also presents with fluctuating muscle weakness. It is the result of autoantibodies against presynaptic voltage-gated calcium channels. 50–60% of patients with LEMS have a tumor as a predisposing factor and small cell lung carcinoma is the most common. Incidence is low (0.48 per million), and patients present with proximal muscle weakness of the limbs that progressively spreads distally in the extremities and cranially in the neck and head. At rest, reflexes are typically absent. Similar to MG, the muscle weakness is variable and after a period of muscle activation weakness and local reflexes are improved. This effect is the opposite of the classic findings in MG.[53]

Clinical examination is paramount in patients with a suspected NMJ disorder. Ptosis or diplopia following sustained upgaze, or the inability to maintain abduction or forward flexion at the shoulder suggests MG. In addition, heightened fatigability with repetitive deltoid exercises also supports this diagnosis. Improvement of ptosis seen following adminis-tration of an ice pack to the eyes is also sensitive and specific for MG. An edrophonium (Tensilon) test also shows improvement in ptosis or ophthalmoparesis in the setting of MG. Conversely, painless weakness of the proximal muscles with hyporeflexia that improves with exercise should raise suspicion for LEMS. Autonomic dysfunction (dry mouth, erectile dysfunction, constipation) may also be seen with LEMS.[54]

Clinical diagnoses of MG and LEMS can be confirmed with laboratory and electrophysiological evaluation. Immunologic assay for acetylcholine receptor antibodies is the first step in evaluation of MG. A negative result would warrant further testing for MuSK and LRP4 antibodies. MG can also be confirmed with repetitive nerve stimulation or single-fiber EMG.[55,56] Diagnosis of LEMS can be confirmed by detection of antibodies against the voltage-gated calcium channel. Nerve conduction studies is characterized by augmentation of CMAP following repetitive nerve stimulation.[53,55]

MUSCULAR DISORDERS

Inflammatory Myopathies

The unifying feature of inflammatory myopathies is immune-mediated muscular injury leading to weakness. Polymyositis (PM) and dermatomyositis (DM) present as idiopathic, progressive symmetric weakness of the proximal limb and trunk muscles. Patients often complain of difficulty performing activities such as climbing stairs, rising from a chair, or combing one's hair. DM is also associated with skin findings such as Gottron's papules, shawl sign, and heliotrope rash. It is common for PM and DM to be associated with other systemic autoimmune diseases such as lupus erythematosus, scleroderma, rheumatoid arthritis, and mixed connective tissue diseases.

Inclusion body myositis is another common form of inflammatory myopathy. Its presentation is typically more variable than PM or DM with symptoms of a progressive, painless muscle weakness that typically manifests distally in the arms, but may also variably affect the proximal and distal lower extremities. DM is the most common form of inflammatory myopathy in all age groups and PM is the rarest. In adults, DM affects persons between the 6th decade and 8th decade of life while PM presents after the 2nd decade of life.[57,58] Both disorders are more prevalent in females.[59] On the other hand, inclusion body myositis is the most prevalent inflammatory myopathy in those older than 50 years.[60] Overall, inflammatory myopathies have an estimated incidence of 2.1–7.7 per million.[58]

Physical exam is useful when inflammatory myopathy is suspected. A thorough skin examination should be performed to exclude DM. Laboratory evaluation will reveal elevated creatine kinase in most cases, but may be normal in inclusion body myopathy. In addition, elevations of aldolase, lactate dehydrogenase, aspartate aminotransferase, alanine aminotransferase, and myoglobin are typical. An autoantibody evaluation is typically performed when an inflammatory myopathy is suspected. These autoantibodies are classified as either myositis-specific autoantibodies (MSA) or myositis-associated autoantibodies (MAA).

Electromyography is also helpful in the diagnosis of inflammatory myopathy and shows abnormalities such as fibrillation potentials, positive sharp waves at rest, and increased insertional activity in 70–90% of patients. However, the findings on EMG are nonspecific and a definitive diagnosis cannot be made on these results alone. Muscle biopsy is the study of choice for a conclusive diagnosis. The muscle chosen for biopsy should be one that has become moderately weak secondary to the disease and each specimen should be evaluated by histochemical staining and immunocytochemistry, which may reveal major histocompatibility complex-1, complement complexes, lymphocytic infiltrates, or vacuoles.[61]

Table 13.2: Muscular dystrophies.

Dystrophy	Muscles affected
Becker muscular dystrophy	Shoulders, hips, quadriceps, calves, and pretibial muscles with pseudohypertrophic calf muscles
Emery-Dreifuss muscular dystrophy	Shoulder and pelvic girdles with possible neck, biceps, and calf contractures
Facioscapulohumeral muscular dystrophy	Shoulder and pelvic girdles with progression to face, chest, and back
Limb-girdle muscular dystrophies	Shoulder and pelvic girdles
Myotonic dystrophy type I	Intrinsic hand muscles, wrist extensors, facial, pharyngeal, laryngeal, and sternocleidomastoids with progression to limbs and trunk
Myotonic dystrophy type I	Proximal lower limb and hand

Muscular Dystrophies

Muscular dystrophies (MD) are progressive, hereditary disorders causing muscle degeneration. Becker muscular dystrophy is a milder, later-onset form of the classic Duchenne muscular dystrophy (DMD). Patients will usually present in their late adolescent to early adult years with progressive paresis in a pattern to similar to DMD—shoulder, hip, quadriceps, calf, and pretibial muscle weakness in the setting of pseudohypertropic calf muscles. Emery-Dreifuss muscular dystrophy (EMD) will present primarily as weakness of the shoulder and pelvic girdles, and will progress distal. Those with EMD may also develop muscle contractures of the neck, biceps, and calves. Myotonic dystrophy type 1 primarily causes weakness of the intrinsic hand muscles, wrist extensors, facial, pharyngeal, laryngeal, and sternocleidomastoids. Progression of this disorder will extend to involvement of the proximal muscles of the limbs as well as the trunk. This disorder is unique in that patients will demonstrate difficulty relaxing following muscle contraction. The spectrum of hereditary MD is extensive and Table 13.2 lists some of the more common pathologies and their affected musculature.

Recognition of the distribution of muscle weakness, atrophy, and pseudohypertrophy will assist in the diagnosis of a muscular dystrophy (Table 13.3). The differential can be narrowed based on this pattern alone. Laboratory studies reveal elevated creatine kinase during the active phase of the disorder, but techniques such as multiplex polymerase chain reaction and genetic testing are necessary to identify the associated chromosomal abnormality, as well as the affected muscular proteins.[62-64] Electromyography studies have classically been used to demonstrate pathognomonic findings of muscle disease.[64] When a diagnosis is unable to be confirmed by less invasive techniques, a muscle biopsy may be necessary. Histologic findings include

Table 13.3: Myotomes.

Myotome level	Major muscle	Major action	Reflex
C5	Deltoid	Abduction of arms > 90° from midline	
C6	Biceps	Forearm flexion and supination	Biceps reflex
C7	Triceps	Forearm extension	Triceps reflex
C8	Most intrinsic hand muscles	Handgrip	
T1	Dorsal interossei	Abduction of fingers	
L2	Iliopsoas	Hip flexion	Cremasteric reflex
L3	Quadriceps	Knee extension	Patellar reflex
L4	Tibialis anterior	Foot dorsiflexion	
L5	Extensor hallucis longus	Big toe extension	
S1	Gastrocnemius and soleus	Foot plantar flexion	Achilles reflex
S2–S4	External anal sphincter	Rectal tone	Anal wink and bulbo-cavernosus reflex

necrotic and regenerating fibers, fiber size variability, and replacement of muscle with fat and connective tissue. Variations in histologic appearance can guide diagnosis. Various antibodies are used during histological analysis to differentiate between muscular dystrophies.[64]

Endocrine Myopathies

Muscle weakness is a common presentation in disorders of the endocrine system, particularly those affecting thyroid hormone or cortisol levels. Thyrotoxic hypokalemic periodic paralysis (THPP) presents as recurrent episodes of severe weakness of the limb and trunk muscles that develops over a few hours and lasts for a day or longer. Proximal muscles are typically more severely affected than distal muscles. These episodes frequently occur following large meals or strenuous exercise.[65]

In THPP, serum thyroid hormone levels may be normal or slightly elevated. The finding of hypokalemia (typically ≤3 mmol/L) is supportive of the diagnosis.[66] The cause of the hypokalemia is a transient intracellular potassium shift and the serum potassium may return to normal following the episode of muscular weakness. The same intracellular shift may also cause a transient hypomagnesemia and hypophosphatemia. EMG recorded during an episode of weakness will demonstrate myopathic changes and NCS will exclude neural etiology. Patients with THPP can also show changes on electrocardiogram (EKG) such as high QRS and a first-degree atrioventricular block.[67]

Abnormal cortisol levels are also causes of muscle weakness. It is estimated that 50–80% of those with Cushing's disease have muscle weakness.[68]

The distribution of weakness is typically proximal, with lower extremities weakened more than the upper extremities. Similarly, glucocorticoid administration is the most common cause of drug-induced myopathy.[69] 24-hour urine cortisol and early AM serum cortisol levels will be elevated during laboratory assessment in the aforementioned settings.

Metabolic Myopathies

Metabolic myopathies represent an extensive topic that will be briefly introduced. Glycogen storage diseases will typically present as painful muscle weakness occurring during exercise, which abates upon resting. Lipid metabolism disorders can present similarly with myalgia, weakness, and stiffness following exercise. The clinical presentation of the various disorders can be quite variable. Evaluation via exercise testing can be utilized in the diagnostic workup. The ischemic forearm exercise test looks at the levels of lactate and ammonia in the venous system following 1 minute of rapid forearm exercise. A similar aerobic exercise test analyzes serum lactate following treadmill use. These tests are simple, minimally-invasive strategies to aid the diagnostician assessing for possible metabolic myopathy. In lieu of positive findings, more invasive techniques such as muscle biopsy with biochemical evaluation are necessary.[70]

CONCLUSION

Generalized progressive paresis may arise from a variety of insults that can target various components of the motor axis. These may include structural, metabolic, and molecular derangements that may have the potential to cause permanent impairment and even death. Treatment response is often time sensitive for entities causing paresis, and it is imperative that appropriate measures be taken early in the course of disease in order to preserve function. The most important tool of an effective diagnostician is the patient's history and physical examination. These elements prompt the clinician to order necessary auxiliary studies to secure the diagnosis, generate treatment plans, and provide a baseline for future follow up. These conditions will come across the desk of almost all physicians at some point in their career, and one must have a good working knowledge of the more emergent and urgent sources of weakness so that proper referrals may be made upon diagnosis.

REFERENCES

1. Adhiyaman V. Chronic subdural haematoma in the elderly. Postgrad Med J. 2002;78(916):71-5.
2. Stiell I, Wells GA, Vandemheen K, et al. The Canadian CT Head Rule for patients with minor head injury. Lancet. 2001;357(9266):1391-6.

3. McKinney PA. Brain tumours: incidence, survival, and aetiology. J Neurol Neurosurg Psychiatry. 2004;75 Suppl 2:ii12-7.

4. Grant R. Overview: brain tumour diagnosis and management/Royal College of Physicians guidelines. J Neurol Neurosurg Psychiatry. 2004;75 Suppl 2:ii18-23.

5. Uchino K, Johnston S, Becker K, et al. Moyamoya disease in Washington State and California. Neurology. 2005;65(6):956-8.

6. Kainth D, Chaudhry S, Kainth H, et al. Epidemiological and clinical features of moyamoya disease in the USA. Neuroepidemiology. 2013;40(4):282-7.

7. Hoffman HJ. Moyamoya disease and syndrome. Clin Neurol Neurosurg. 1997;99 Suppl 2:S39-44.

8. Starke R, Komotar R, Hickman Z, et al. Clinical features, surgical treatment, and long-term outcome in adult patients with moyamoya disease. J Neurosurg. 2009;111(5):936-42.

9. Deng X, Wang K, Wu L, et al. Asymmetry of tonsillar ectopia, syringomyelia and clinical manifestations in adult Chiari I malformation. Acta Neurochir (Wein). 2014;156(4):715-22.

10. Koehler P. Chiari's description of cerebellar ectopy (1891) with a summary of Cleland's and Arnold's contributions and some early observations on neural-tube defects. J Neurosurg. 1991;75(5):823-6.

11. Speer M, Enterline D, Mehltretter L, et al. Review article: Chiari type I malformation with or without syringomyelia: Prevalence and genetics. J Genet Couns. 2003;12(4):297-311.

12. Tubbs R, Lyerly M, Loukas M, et al. The pediatric Chiari I malformation: a review. Childs Nerv Syst. 2007;23(11):1239-50.

13. Hofkes S, Iskandar B, Turski P, et al. Differentiation between Symptomatic Chiari I Malformation and Asymptomatic Tonsilar Ectopia by Using Cerebrospinal Fluid Flow Imaging: Initial Estimate of Imaging Accuracy 1. Radiology. 2007;245(2):532-40.

14. Konno S, Meyer J, Terayama Y, et al. Classification, Diagnosis and Treatment of Vascular Dementia. Drugs Aging. 1997;11(5):361-73.

15. Apostolova LG, DeKosky ST, Cummings JL. Dementias. In: Daroff RB, Fenichel GM, Jankovic J, Mazziotta JC (Eds). Bradley's Neurology in Clinical Practice, 6th edition. Philadelphia, PA: Elsevier Saunders; 2012.

16. Moorhouse PA, Rockwood K. Vascular cognitive impairment. In: Fillit HM, Rockwood K, Woodhouse K (Eds). Brocklehurst's Textbook of Geriatric Medicine and Gerontology, 7th edition. Philadelphia, PA; 2010.

17. Kaplin AI, Krishnan C, Deshpande DM, et al. Diagnosis and management of acute myelopathies. Neurologist. 2005;11(1):2-18.

18. Beh SC, Greenberg BM, Frohman T, et al. Transverse myelitis. Neurol Clin. 2013;31(1):79-138.

19. Polman CH, Reingold SC, Banwell B, et al. Diagnostic criteria for multiple sclerosis: 2010 revisions to the McDonald criteria. Ann Neurol. 2011;69(2):292-302.

20. Kampman MT, Brustad M. Vitamin D: a candidate for the environmental effect in multiple sclerosis - observations from Norway. Neuroepidemiology. 2008;30(3):140-6.

21. Filippi M, Rocca MA. MR imaging of multiple sclerosis. Radiology. 2011;259 (3):659-81.

22. Drori T, Chapman J. Diagnosis and classification of neuromyelitis optica (Devic's syndrome). Autoimmun Rev. 2014;13(4-5):531-3.

23. Katz JN. Lumbar spinal fusion. Surgical rates, costs, and complications. Spine. 1995;15(20):78S-83S.

24. Katz JN, Harris MB. Clinical practice. Lumbar spinal stenosis. New Engl J Med. 2008;358(8):818-25.

25. Bernhardt M, Hynes RA, Blume HW, et al. Cervical spondylotic myelopathy. J Bone Joint Surg Am. 1993;75(1):119-28.

26. Teresi L, Lufkin R, Reicher M, et al. Asymptomatic degenerative disk disease and spondylosis of the cervical spine: MR imaging. Radiology. 1987;164(1):83-8.

27. Katz JN, Dalgas M, Stucki G, et al. Degenerative lumbar spinal stenosis. Diagnostic value of the history and physical examination. Arthritis Rheum. 1995;38(9):1236-41.

28. Crandall PH, Batzdorf U. Cervical spondylotic myelopathy. J Neurosurg. 1966;25(1):57-66.

29. Chou R, Qaseem A, Owens DK, et al. Diagnostic imaging for low back pain: advice for high-value health care from the American College of Physicians. Ann Intern Med. 2011;154(3):181-9.

30. Hall S, Bartleson JD, Onofrio BM, et al. Lumbar spinal stenosis. Clinical features, diagnostic procedures, and results of surgical treatment in 68 patients. Ann Intern Med. 1985;103(2):271-5.

31. de Graaf I, Prak A, Bierma-Zeinstra S, et al. Diagnosis of lumbar spinal stenosis: a systematic review of the accuracy of diagnostic tests. Spine. 2006;31(10):1168-76.

32. Soehle M, Wallenfang T. Spinal epidural abscesses: clinical manifestations, prognostic factors, and outcomes. Neurosurgery. 2002;51(1):79-87.

33. Darouiche RO. Spinal epidural abscess. New Engl J Med. 2006;355(19):2012-20.

34. Grewal S, Hocking G, Wildsmith JA. Epidural abscesses. Br J Anaesth. 2006;96(3):292-302.

35. Patsalides A, Santillan A, Knopman J, et al. Endovascular management of spinal dural arteriovenous fistulas. J Neurointerv Surg. 2011;3(1):80-4.

36. Anson JA, Spetzler RF. Interventional neuroradiology for spinal pathology. Clin Neurosurg. 1992;39:388-417.

37. Krings T. Vascular malformations of the spine and spinal cord*: anatomy, classification, treatment. Clin Neuroradiol. 2010;20(1):5-24.

38. Narvid J, Hetts SW, Larsen D, et al. Spinal dural arteriovenous fistulae: clinical features and long-term results. Neurosurgery. 2008;62(1):159-67.

39. Lev N, Maimon S, Rappaport ZH, et al. Spinal dural arteriovenous fistulae--a diagnostic challenge. Isr Med Assoc J. 2001;3(7):492-6.

40. Saraf-Lavi E, Bowen BC, Quencer RM, et al. Detection of spinal dural arteriovenous fistulae with MR imaging and contrast-enhanced MR angiography: sensitivity, specificity, and prediction of vertebral level. AJNR Am J Neuroradiol. 2002;23(5):858-67.

41. Prasad D, Schiff D. Malignant spinal-cord compression. Lancet Oncol. 2005;6(1):15-24.

42. Chamberlain MC, Tredway TL. Adult primary intradural spinal cord tumors: a review. Current Neurol Neurosci Rep. 2011;11(3):320-8.

43. Schiff D, O'Neill BP. Intramedullary spinal cord metastases: clinical features and treatment outcome. Neurology. 1996;47(4):906-12.

44. Traul D, Shaffrey M, Schiff D. Part I: Spinal-cord neoplasms—intradural neoplasms. Lancet Oncol. 2007;8(1):35-45.

45. Sreedharan J, Brown RH. Amyotrophic lateral sclerosis: Problems and prospects. Ann Neurol. 2013;74(3):309-16.

46. de Carvalho M, Dengler R, Eisen A, et al. Electrodiagnostic criteria for diagnosis of ALS. Clin Neurophysiol. 2008;119(3):497-503.

47. Vucic S, Kiernan MC, Cornblath DR. Guillain-Barré syndrome: an update. J Clin Neurosci. 2009;16(6):733-41.

48. Hughes RA, Cornblath DR. Guillain-Barré syndrome. Lancet. 2005;366(9497): 1653-66.

49. Thadani H, Deacon A, Peters T. Diagnosis and management of porphyria. BMJ. 2000;320(7250):1647-51.

50. Köller H, Kieseier BC, Jander S, et al. Chronic inflammatory demyelinating polyneuropathy. N Engl J Med. 2005;352(13):1343-56.

51. Carr AS, Cardwell CR, McCarron PO, et al. A systematic review of population based epidemiological studies in Myasthenia Gravis. BMC Neurol. 2010;10(1):46.

52. Meriggioli MN, Sanders DB. Autoimmune myasthenia gravis: emerging clinical and biological heterogeneity. Lancet Neurol. 2009;8(5):475-90.

53. Titulaer MJ, Lang B, Verschuuren JJ. Lambert-Eaton myasthenic syndrome: from clinical characteristics to therapeutic strategies. Lancet Neurol. 2011;10(12):1098-107.

54. Reddy AR, Backhouse OC. "Ice-on-eyes", a simple test for myasthenia gravis presenting with ocular symptoms. Pract Neurol. 2007;7(2):109-11.

55. Liang CL, Han S. Neuromuscular junction disorders. PM R. 2013;5(5 Suppl): S81-8.

56. Berrih-Aknin S, Frenkian-Cuvelier M, Eymard B. Diagnostic and clinical classification of autoimmune myasthenia gravis. J Autoimmun. 2014;48-49:143-8.

57. Iaccarino L, Ghirardello A, Bettio S, et al. The clinical features, diagnosis and classification of dermatomyositis. J Autoimmun. 2014;48-49:122-7.

58. Milisenda JC, Selva-O'Callaghan A, Grau JM. The diagnosis and classification of polymyositis. J Autoimmun. 2014;48-49:118-21.

59. Khan S, Christopher-Stine L. Polymyositis, dermatomyositis, and autoimmune necrotizing myopathy: clinical features. Rheum Dis Clin North Am. 2011;37(2):143-58.

60. Catalán M, Selva-O'Callaghan A, Grau JM. Diagnosis and classification of sporadic inclusion body myositis (sIBM). Autoimmun Rev. 2014;13(4-5):363-6.

61. Dalakas MC. Review: An update on inflammatory and autoimmune myopathies. Neuropathol Appl Neurobiol. 2011;37(3):226-42.

62. Selva-O'Callaghan A, Trallero-Araguás E, Grau JM. Eosinophilic myositis: an updated review. Autoimmun Rev. 2014;13(4-5):375-8.

63. Flanigan KM. The muscular dystrophies. Semin Neurol. 2012;32(3):255-63.

64. Shieh PB. Muscular dystrophies and other genetic myopathies. Neurol Clin. 2013;31(4):1009-29.

65. Mercuri E, Muntoni F. Muscular dystrophies. Lancet. 2013;381(9869):845-60.

66. Kung AW. Clinical review: Thyrotoxic periodic paralysis: a diagnostic challenge. J Clin Endocrinol Metab. 2006;91(7):2490-5.

67. Hsu YJ, Lin YF, Chau T, et al. Electrocardiographic manifestations in patients with thyrotoxic periodic paralysis. Am J Med Sci. 2003;326(3):128-32.

68. Urbanic RC, George JM. Cushing's disease--18 years' experience. Medicine (Baltimore). 1981;60(1):14-24.

69. Pereira RM, Freire de Carvalho J. Glucocorticoid-induced myopathy. Joint Bone Spine. 2011;78(1):41-4.

70. Volpi L, Ricci G, Orsucci D, et al. Metabolic myopathies: functional evaluation by different exercise testing approaches. Musculoskelet Surg. 2011;95(2):59-67.

CHAPTER 14

MRI Cord Changes

Vahe M Zohrabian, Adam E Flanders

INTRODUCTION

Myelopathy refers to any neurological deficit related to dysfunction of the spinal cord, and can be acute or chronic. Although there are myriad of causes, myelopathy is most frequently due to cord compression in the setting of disk disease, extradural metastases, or blunt/penetrating trauma. Less commonly, intrinsic cord lesions may result in myelopathy, and include, but are not limited to, inflammatory, infectious, and neoplastic etiologies. Magnetic resonance imaging (MRI) is the test of choice for myelopathy given its ability to directly visualize the spinal canal and neural structures. MRI allows for prompt recognition of abnormal spinal cord signal and morphology, and the information obtained, in combination with the clinical history, aids in accurate diagnosis and the potential to reverse damage. Here, we focus on several common spinal cord diseases that are characterized by high signal in the cord on T2-weighted MRI, and categorize them into inflammatory, neoplastic, vascular, metabolic, and traumatic causes. A brief patient history is offered at the beginning of each section to allow for an appropriate differential diagnosis.

INFLAMMATORY CAUSES

Chief complaint/history: A 31-year-old white female with long-term neurologic complaints, including bilateral hand numbness, heat intolerance, and decreased visual acuity.

Differential diagnosis:
• Multiple sclerosis (MS)
• Idiopathic acute transverse myelitis (IATM)
• Lupus myelitis.

Discussion:
Multiple sclerosis is a common, chronic, inflammatory demyelinating disease of the central nervous system. MS plaques are characteristically perivenous,

with early lesions, or "active" plaques, demonstrating lymphocytes and macrophages.[1] In the subacute stage, lymphocytes are replaced by macrophages, while chronic, or "inactive," lesions are characterized by gliosis and cavitation.[1] Typically affecting young to middle-aged females, concomitant brain and spinal cord involvement is far more common than isolated spinal cord disease.[2,3] The cervical segment of the spinal cord, especially the dorsolateral cord, is most commonly affected.[4] On MRI, MS "plaques" present as focal, ovoid, peripherally located asymmetric areas of T2-hyperintensity elongated in the direction of the long axis of the cord and not respecting gray-white matter boundaries. These plaques are usually less than two vertebral body segments in length and occupy less than half the cross-sectional area of the spinal cord[3,5] (Figs. 14.1A and B). On axial sequences, MS lesions are characteristically wedge shaped with their apices directed centrally (Fig. 14.1C). These plaques are rarely visible as discrete hypointense foci on T1-weighted images, usually appearing T1-isointense. Short tau inversion recovery (STIR) sequences can increase sensitivity for lesion detection.[6] The cord is typically normal in caliber, although rarely, there may be mild enlargement due to edema. On post-gadolinium sequences, MS plaques may show homogeneous,

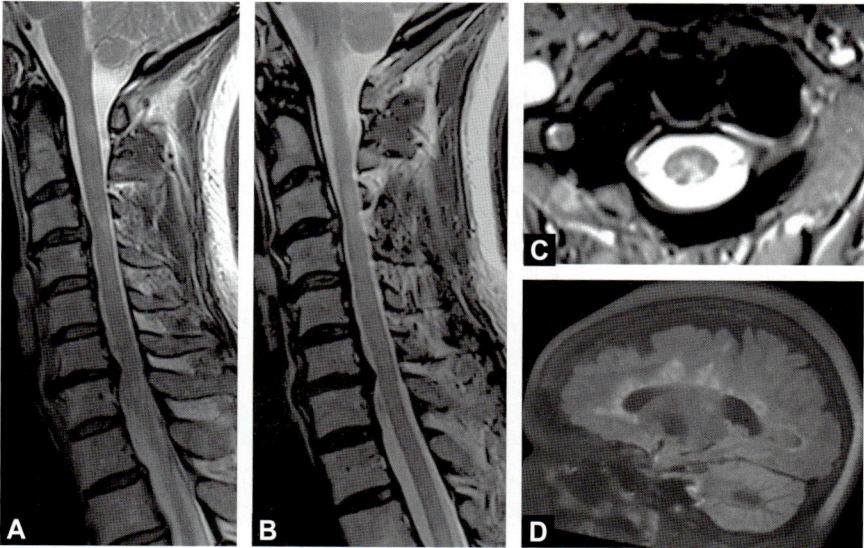

Figs. 14.1A to D: Multiple sclerosis. (A) Sagittal T2WI of the cervical spine demonstrates focal, short segment intramedullary hyperintensities measuring less than 2 vertebral body segments in length at the top of C2 and at the C3-C4 level, (B) sagittal T2WI from the same patient demonstrates a discrete, ovoid well-defined intramedullary hyperintensity at the level of C2-C3, and subtle hyperintensity at the T2 level, (C) axial T2WI shows abnormal signal involving both central gray and dorsolateral white matter. There is no cord expansion, (D) a sagittal fluid-attenuated inversion recovery (FLAIR) image from the same patient's brain MRI reveals numerous periventricular T2-hyperintensities arranged perpendicular to the lateral ventricles and extending radially outward (Dawson fingers).

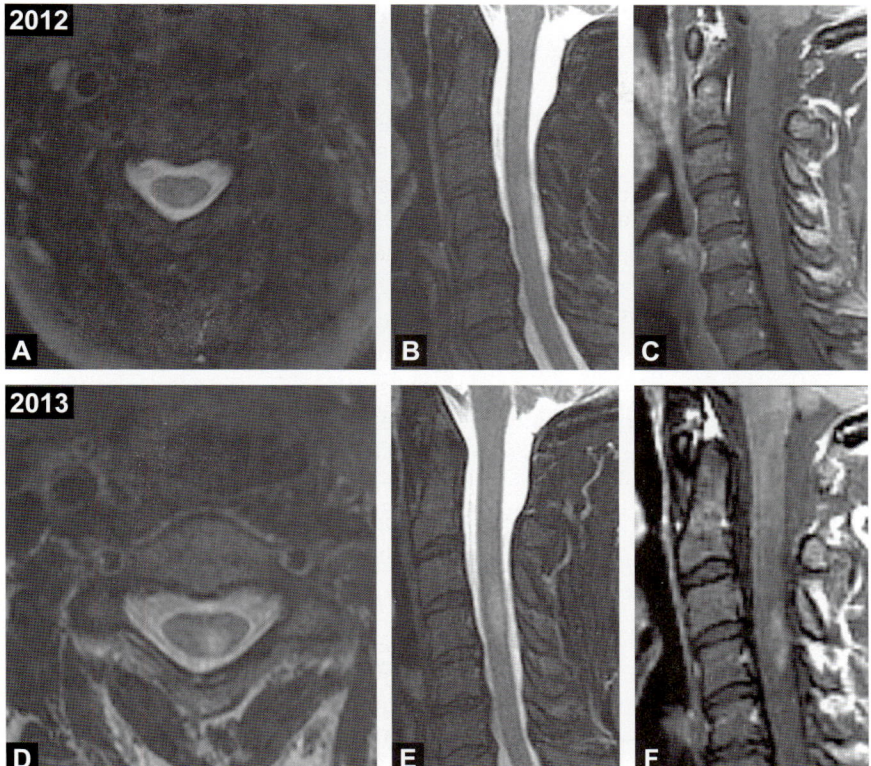

Figs. 14.2A to F: Dissemination in time. (A and B) Axial and sagittal short tau inversion recovery (STIR) in a patient with multiple sclerosis demonstrates subtle, short segment intramedullary hyperintensity in the dorsolateral cord at the C4 level, (C) post-gadolinium T1WI reveals no enhancement in association with this lesion, (D and E) axial T2WI and sagittal STIR from the same patient performed 1 year later demonstrates interval increase in conspicuity of the lesion centered at C4, (F) post-gadolinium T1WI reveals enhancement associated with this lesion, compatible with active disease/demyelination.

nodular, or peripheral enhancement in the acute or subacute phases. In chronic MS, there may be generalized cord thinning/atrophy, which has been associated with greater disability.[7] If a patient is suspected of MS based on spinal cord findings, it is recommended to image the brain to look for white matter abnormalities, with special attention to the sagittal fluid-attenuated inversion recovery (FLAIR) sequence (Fig. 14.1D). However, it is important to keep in mind that a negative brain MRI does not exclude MS.[2] Moreover, as the hallmark of MS is multiple lesions disseminated over time and space, signal abnormalities may appear or disappear on consecutive studies (Figs. 14.2A to F).

Transverse myelitis (TM) refers to an inflammatory disorder of the spinal cord secondary to a multitude of causes, including but not limited to, demyelinating disorders, viral or bacterial infections, connective tissue

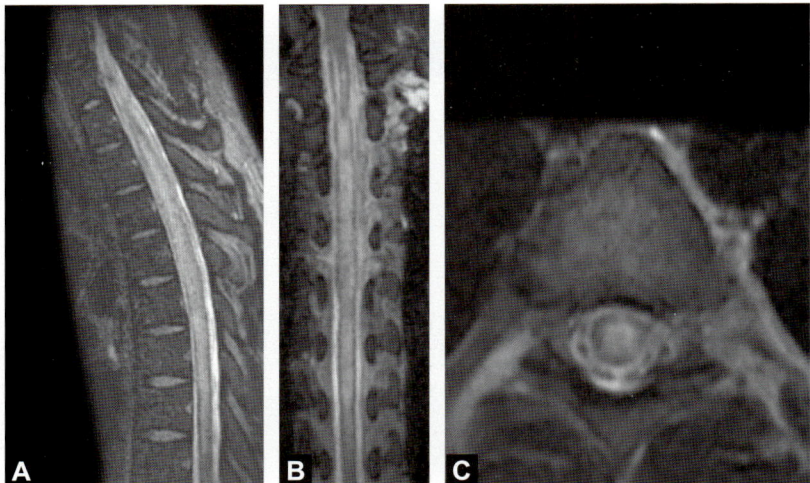

Figs. 14.3A to C: Transverse myelitis. (A) Sagittal short tau inversion recovery (STIR), (B) coronal STIR, and (C) axial T2WI demonstrate long segment central T2-hyperintensity in the cervicothoracic cord occupying greater than two-thirds the cross-sectional area of the cord and resulting in mild, smooth cord expansion.

diseases, sarcoidosis, radiotherapy, and Behcet syndrome. When there is no identifiable cause, the disease is termed "idiopathic acute transverse myelitis," which is usually monophasic. MRI of IATM demonstrates central T2-hyperintensity occupying more than two-thirds the cross-sectional area of the spinal cord, typically in the thoracic region, and extending greater than 2 (~3–4) vertebral body segments in length. There is usually smooth, symmetric cord expansion[8] (Figs. 14.3A to C). Post-gadolinium sequences may show enhancement, which can be both patchy and diffuse (Table 14.1). A special note is made of lupus myelitis, a recognized complication of systemic lupus erythematosus (SLE) primarily affecting females. MRI in lupus myelitis demonstrates central increased T2-signal occupying more than two-thirds the cross-sectional area of the cord and extending greater than 3–4 vertebral body segments in length, along with variable, inconsistent enhancement.[9,10]

Neuromyelitis optica (NMO), or Devic syndrome, is an autoimmune, inflammatory mono- or multiphasic demyelinating disease distinct from MS induced by the autoantibody NMO-IgG, which is directed against the aquaporin-4 water channel. NMO preferentially affects the optic nerves and spinal cord, and usually has a more rapid, debilitating course than MS. On MRI, NMO is similar in appearance to IATM, characterized by longitudinal, confluent, long segment (>=3 vertebral bodies) T2-hyperintensity involving the entire cross-sectional area of the cord (Fig. 14.4A). There may be cord swelling and/or enhancement (Figs. 14.4B and C), along with enhancement of the optic nerves (optic neuritis) (Fig. 14.4D). Although there is limited brain involvement, periventricular white matter lesions can be seen.

Table 14.1: MS versus IATM.

MS	IATM
Cervical more common	Typically thoracic
Short, < 2 vertebral segments in length	Longer, ~3–4 segments in length
< 1/2 cross-sectional area of cord	> 2/3 cord cross-sectional area
90% associated intracranial lesions	No associated intracranial lesions

(MS: Multiple sclerosis; IATM: Idiopathic acute transverse myelitis).

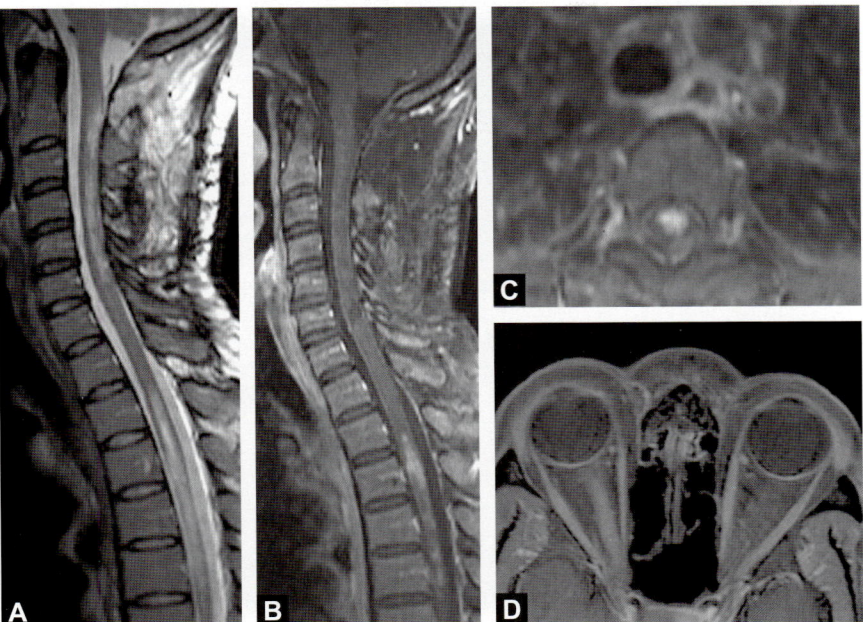

Figs. 14.4A to D: Neuromyelitis optica. (A) Sagittal T2WI reveals long-segment cord enlargement and T2 hyperintensity from C2-C6 and T2-T6, (B and C) post-gadolinium sagittal and axial T1WI demonstrate associated enhancement in the upper thoracic cord from T2/T3 to T5/T6, (D) MRI of the optic nerves in the same patient shows marked enhancement of the intraorbital and intracanalicular segments of the right optic nerve. Acute myelopathy and optic neuritis may occur at the same time, although is usually separated by days.

Acute disseminated encephalomyelitis (ADEM) is an uncommon, immune-mediated widespread demyelinating disorder affecting the brain, and less frequently, the spinal cord. More common in pediatric patients, the symptoms of ADEM usually develop within a few weeks after the onset of a viral infection or vaccination.[11] ADEM is typically monophasic, in contrast to MS; however, recurrent or multiphasic forms have been reported.[12] MRI shows punctate to segmental multifocal T2-hyperintensities anywhere in the spinal cord white or gray matter with little mass effect or edema, along with slight cord expansion (Figs. 14.5A to C). The thoracic segment of the cord is

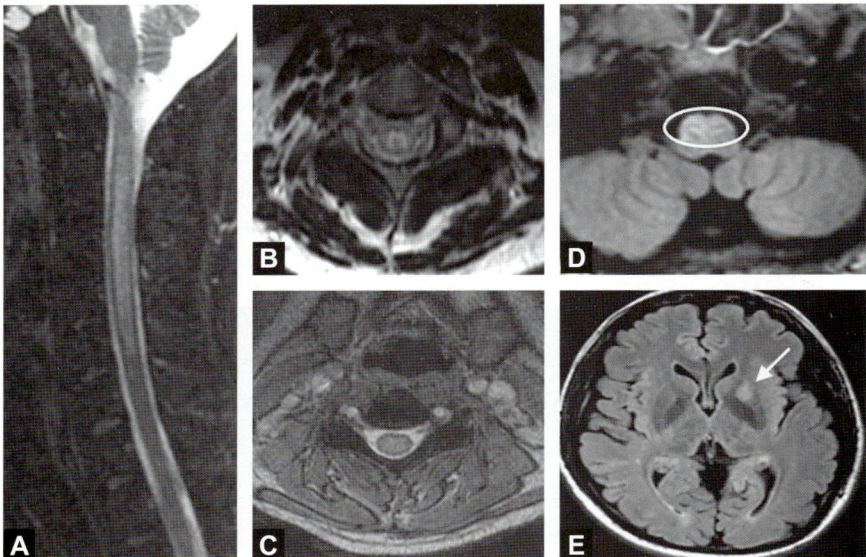

Figs. 14.5A to E: Acute disseminated encephalomyelitis. (A) Sagittal short tau inversion recovery (STIR) demonstrates long-segment intramedullary hyperintensity spanning C2 to C5/C6 with mild, smooth cord expansion, (B and C) axial T2WI and gradient-echo sequence also reveals abnormal intramedullary signal, (D) axial fluid-attenuated inversion recovery (FLAIR) from brain MRI in the same patient at the level of the posterior fossa/lower brain stem shows increased signal in the anterior medulla (oval), (E) FLAIR image more cranially shows focal increased signal in the left putamen (arrow).

most frequently affected in ADEM.[12] Post-gadolinium sequences demonstrate variable punctate, ring-shaped, or fluffy enhancement. There may also be involvement of the peripheral nervous system, as manifested by abnormal cranial nerve enhancement; as such, ADEM cannot be differentiated from NMO at first presentation. Brain MRI reveals multifocal white matter and deep gray lesions, which may be mass-like, and the brain stem and posterior fossa can be involved (Figs. 14.5D and E). If the MRI is initially negative, patients suspected of ADEM should be reimaged since there may be a delay between the onset of clinical symptoms and imaging findings.

NEOPLASTIC CAUSES

Chief complaint/history: A 42-year-old male with a 4-week history of progressive back pain, weakness in both lower limbs, and difficulty urinating.

Differential diagnosis:
- Spinal cord neoplasm
- Demyelinating disease
- Dural vascular malformation.

Discussion:

Spinal cord tumors may be intramedullary or extramedullary, and are classified as primary or secondary. Ependymoma and astrocytoma are the two most common primary intramedullary tumors, with ependymoma representing the most common tumor of the lower spinal cord, conus medullaris, and filum terminale. Typically affecting middle-aged males,[13] ependymomas arise from cells lining the central canal of the spinal cord, and as such, are usually well-circumscribed, central masses resulting in fairly symmetric cord expansion. On MRI, ependymomas are usually well-defined, isointense/ hypointense to spinal cord on T1-weighted sequences, and heterogeneous on T2-weighted images. It is sometimes possible to delineate a subtle cleavage plane between the tumor and the cord. Furthermore, although calcification is rare, hemorrhage (T1-hyperintensity) is common, as is T1- and marked T2-hypointense hemosiderin deposition at the cranial and/or caudal ends of the tumor, resulting in the so-called "cap sign". Moreover, intratumoral cysts lined by abnormal glial cells, benign rostral or caudal cysts (polar cysts), and/or syrinx secondary to partial obstruction are not infrequent. Gadolinium enhancement is intense yet irregular/heterogeneous. Gadolinium is also helpful in distinguishing intratumoral cysts, which demonstrate peripheral wall enhancement, from polar cysts and syrinx, which do not enhance.[14] Myxopapillary ependymomas, a particular subtype of ependymoma, are intradural extramedullary masses that are usually isointense on T1- and hyperintense on T2-weighted sequences, although may demonstrate alternate signal characteristics in the setting of calcification and/or hemorrhage (Figs. 14.6A to D). Given that they are prone to hemorrhage, it is important to image the lower spine in the setting of unexplained subarachnoid hemorrhage to exclude a myxopapillary ependymoma.[15]

Astrocytomas occur mostly in children and young to middle-aged adults, with a slight male predominance, and are typically found in the cervical or upper thoracic spine.[16,17] Astrocytomas, unlike ependymomas, are infiltrative and arise eccentrically in the spinal cord, usually in its posterior aspect. These tumors result in fusiform cord expansion and may extend over multiple segments. The pilocytic subtype involves the entire cord. Astrocytomas are less often hemorrhagic and hypervascular compared with ependymomas. On MRI, these lesions are isointense/hypointense on T1- and hyperintense on T2-weighted sequences, and are more often homogeneous when compared with ependymomas. Given their infiltrative nature, however, they may be hard to distinguish from edema in the adjacent cord. Astrocytomas may also demonstrate intratumoral cysts, as well as benign rostral or caudal cysts, which can be isointense to hyperintense on T1-weighted sequences secondary to proteinaceous or hemorrhagic components[18] (Figs. 14.7A to C). Although gadolinium enhancement is nearly always present in astrocytomas, it is often variable when compared with ependymomas (Fig. 14.7D and Table 14.2).

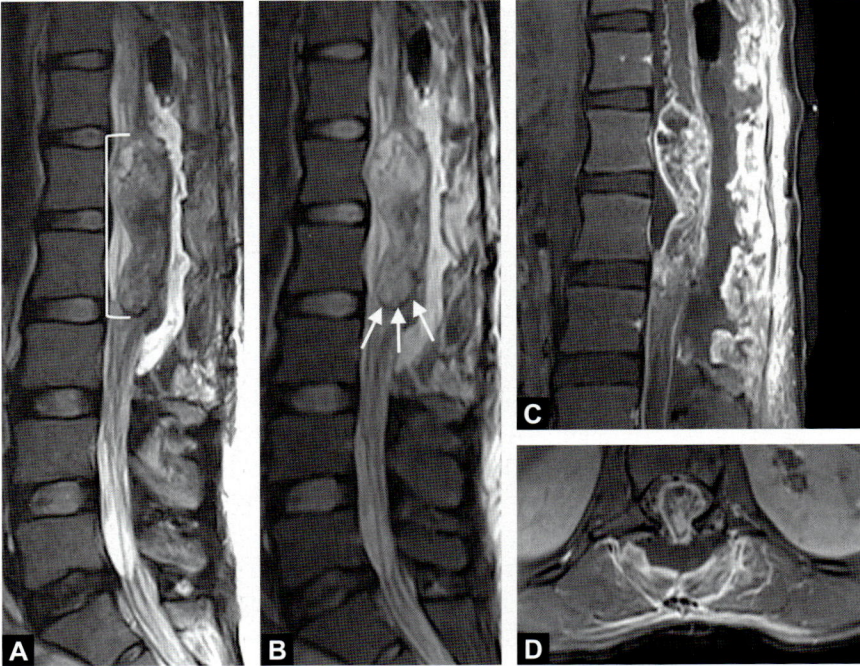

Figs. 14.6A to D: Myxopapillary ependymoma. (A and B) Sagittal T2WI and short tau inversion recovery (STIR) reveals a recurrent large, heterogeneous mass centered in the conus medullaris, measuring up to approximately 7.5 cm in craniocaudal dimension, in this postoperative patient. There is mild widening of the spinal canal. T2-hypointense hemosiderin capping is noted at the inferior pole of the mass (arrows), (C and D) post-gadolinium sagittal and axial T1WI reveals intense, heterogeneous enhancement of the mass, as well as prominent leptomeningeal enhancement above and below the mass.

Hemangioblastomas rarely involve the spinal cord. Multiple hemangioblastomas may be seen in patients with von Hippel-Lindau disease. These tumors are typically intramedullary, although may occasionally be intradural extramedullary or extradural. Hemangioblastomas are most common in the thoracic cord, followed by the cervical cord.[19] The MRI hallmark of a hemangioblastoma is a subpial mass in the posterior aspect of the cord with intraspinal cysts that are of varied signal intensity secondary to proteinaceous or hemorrhagic fluid. The post-gadolinium sequences demonstrate a small, intensely and uniformly enhancing solid nodule with marked T1-hypointense, T2-hyperintense edema in the surrounding cord.[20] Furthermore, hemangioblastomas may demonstrate intratumoral T2-hypointense flow voids or enhancing serpiginous areas, along with prominent posterior draining veins, allowing its differentiation from cord metastases given that both may show considerable edema surrounding an avidly enhancing solid nodule.[21]

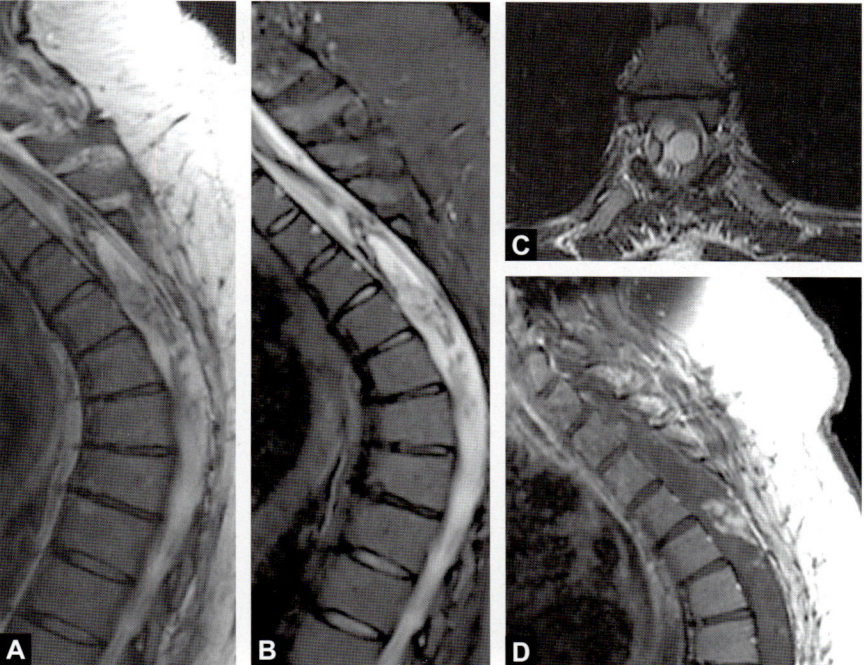

Figs. 14.7A to D: Astrocytoma. (A to C) Sagittal T2WI, sagittal short tau inversion recovery (STIR), and axial T2WI demonstrate a heterogeneous, multicystic intramedullary mass in the midthoracic cord. Areas of T2-hypointense hemosiderin staining are noted, (D) post-gadolinium sagittal T1WI reveals associated irregular enhancement.

Table 14.2: Ependymoma versus astrocytoma.

Ependymoma	Astrocytoma
Middle-aged, male	Children to young adults, male
Lower cord, conus (myxopapillary)	Cervical, upper thoracic
Well-circumscribed, heterogeneous	Infiltrative, homogenous
Central	Eccentric
Hemorrhage common	Less often hemorrhagic
Intense, irregular enhancement	Variable enhancement

Intramedullary cord metastases are rare, with lung cancer accounting for most cases. Metastases reach the spinal cord by arterial seeding, the vertebral venous system, or direct invasion from the nerve roots/cerebrospinal fluid (CSF). Most common in the thoracic cord, metastases result in cord expansion and significant T2-hyperintense edema out of proportion to the size of the small nidus on MRI (Fig. 14.8A). Unlike hemangioblastomas, there is no association with cysts or a syrinx. The metastatic deposit is usually hypointense on T2-weighted sequences, and post-gadolinium sequences

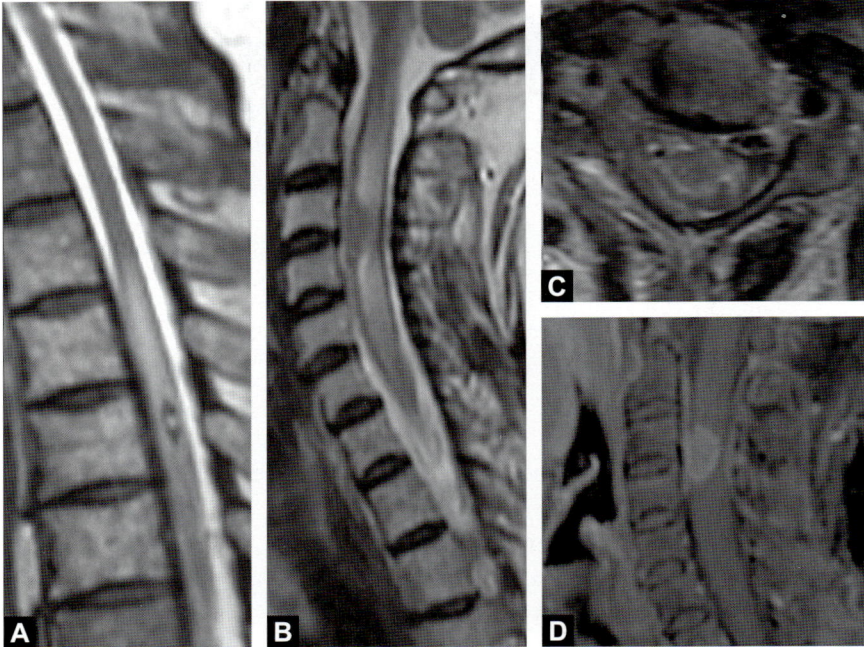

Figs. 14.8A to D: Cord metastases. (A) Sagittal T2WI demonstrates a targetoid, 9 mm, well-circumscribed mixed T2 signal lesion at T5 with considerable surrounding T2-hyperintense edema in this patient with renal cell carcinoma, (B to D) sagittal T2WI, axial T2WI, and post-gadolinium sagittal T1WI in a different patient with breast carcinoma reveals a well-defined T2-hypointense lesion in the anterolateral aspect of the cord at C3-C4 with homogenous enhancement and surrounding reactive edema.

typically demonstrate marked, homogeneous enhancement (Figs. 14.8B to D). Hemorrhage within these lesions is rare.

VASCULAR CAUSES

Chief complaint/history: A 64-year-old male with sudden onset of paraplegia, as well as loss of bowel and bladder continence, after an episode of severe chest pain. There is no history of fever or trauma.

Differential diagnosis:
- Spinal cord ischemia/infarction
- Spinal cord injury (SCI)
- Disk herniation.

Discussion:
The anterior spinal artery (ASA), which supplies approximately two-thirds of the entire cross-sectional area of the spinal cord, courses along the ventral surface of the cord and receives contributions from radicular artery

branches at various locations, known as "radiculomedullary" arteries. The smaller paired posterior spinal arteries (PSAs) course along the dorsal surface of the cord, receive contributions from radiculopial branches of the radicular arteries, and supply most of the posterior white matter tracts. Although communications exist between the PSAs, there are no reliable anastomoses between the territories of the ASA and PSAs. The ASA axis can be divided into three zones, with hemodynamic watershed areas occurring at the margins of these zones, as follows: (1) cervicothoracic, (2) midthoracic, and (3) thoracolumbar. The thoracolumbar region, which extends from T8 through the conus medullaris, receives rich blood supply through a single, large radiculomedullary artery, known as the artery of Adamkiewicz, which usually enters the spinal canal from T9 through T12 on the left.

Spinal cord infarction is most commonly the result of hypotension affecting the ASA or compromise of a radiculomedullary vessel, usually in the setting of aortic pathology, such as surgery, atherosclerosis, and aneurysm. On MRI, cord infarction commonly presents as nonspecific, intrinsic T2-hyperintensity (Fig. 14.9A), with more severe cases affecting both gray and white matter, and therefore, suggesting both ASA and PSA involvement. In the acute stage, the cord may be enlarged or tumor-like on T1-weighted sequences. Furthermore, diffusion-weighted sequences, much like in the brain, can be useful (Fig. 14.9B). The classic teaching is intramedullary abnormal signal in the central cord on axial sequences involving the gray matter in an "owl's eye" pattern (Fig. 14.9C). Post-gadolinium sequences may demonstrate enhancement, especially of the central gray matter, which can last for several months. Moreover, T2-hyperintense areas of infarction in adjacent vertebral bodies may aid in the diagnosis[22] (Fig. 14.9D).

Spinal dural arteriovenous fistula (SDAVF) is the most common spinal arteriovenous malformation (AVM) (type I AVM). Unlike the abrupt onset of symptoms seen with cord infarction, SDAVF presents as a slowly progressive myelopathy, which may be worsened by exercise, usually affecting males in their 5th or 6th decade. The nidus is located inside the dura of the nerve root sleeve, where a single radiculomeningeal artery enters a radicular vein, resulting in engorgement of spinal pial veins, most prominent along the dorsal surface of the cord.[23] The increased venous pressure (venous hypertension) is transmitted to intrinsic veins of the cord, and results in decreased arteriovenous pressure gradient with tissue hypoxia and edema. In the chronic stages, it is associated with progressive "subacute necrotizing myelopathy", referred to as Foix-Alajouanine syndrome.[24,25] Although spinal angiography remains the gold standard in the diagnosis of SDAVF, MRI is critical. MRI may demonstrate nonspecific, abnormal intramedullary T2-hyperintensity representing venous hypertension, most commonly at

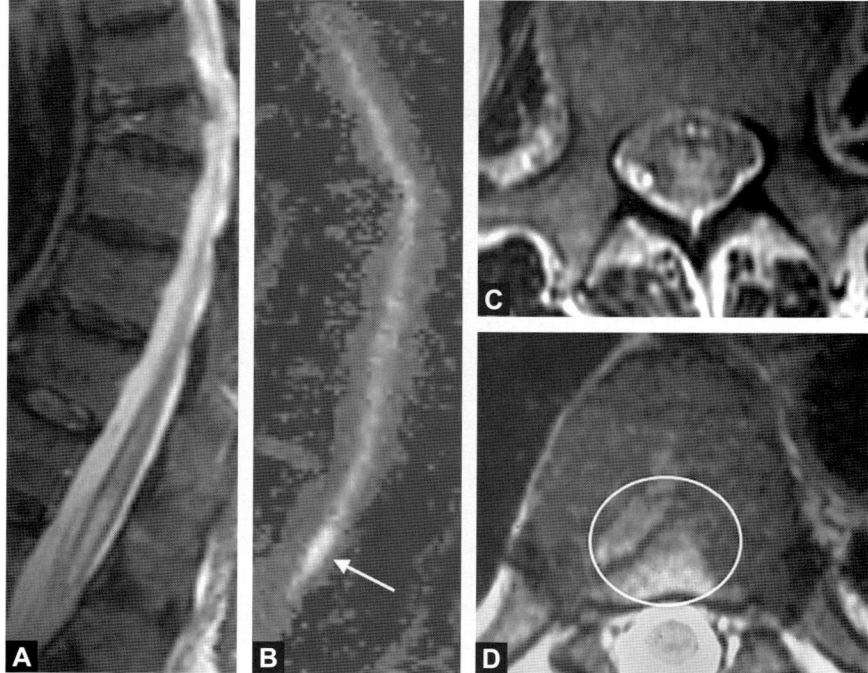

Figs. 14.9A to D: Spinal cord infarct. (A) Sagittal short tau inversion recovery (STIR) demonstrates abnormal T2-hyperintensity in the lower thoracic cord/conus medullaris with mild, smooth cord expansion in this 72-year-old male with sudden onset of paraplegia, (B) diffusion sequence reveals increased signal most suggestive of an acute cord infarct (arrow), (C) axial T2WI demonstrates abnormal hyperintensity in the cord in a classic "owl's eye" pattern, (D) axial T2WI in a different patient with cord infarction reveals abnormal, wedge-shaped T2-hyperintense signal in the posterior aspect of the vertebral body (circle), suggestive of a partial vertebral body infarct in the distribution of the posterior central arteries arising from the spinal branch of the segmental artery.

the level of the conus medullaris (Fig. 14.10A); however, abnormal signal may extend to the level of the upper thoracic spine. Furthermore, T2-hypo-intensity in the cord periphery has been described as an imaging feature of venous hypertensive myelopathy in the setting of SDAVF.[26] The cord may be normal in size or expanded. Hemorrhage is extremely rare. There may also be patchy, ill-defined enhancement within the substance of the spinal cord in the setting of venous hypertension. Most specific for the diagnosis, although not always present, is dilated pial veins, most prominent along the dorsal surface of the cord, and best appreciated on sagittal T2-weighted sequences as tiny areas of flow-void in a background of hyperintense CSF (Fig. 14.10A). The posterior aspect of the spinal cord is normally smooth. It is important not to confuse this appearance with CSF flow-related artifacts, and therefore, the administration of gadolinium is useful in demonstrating enhancing, engorged pial veins (Fig. 14.10B). A type II spinal AVM, or

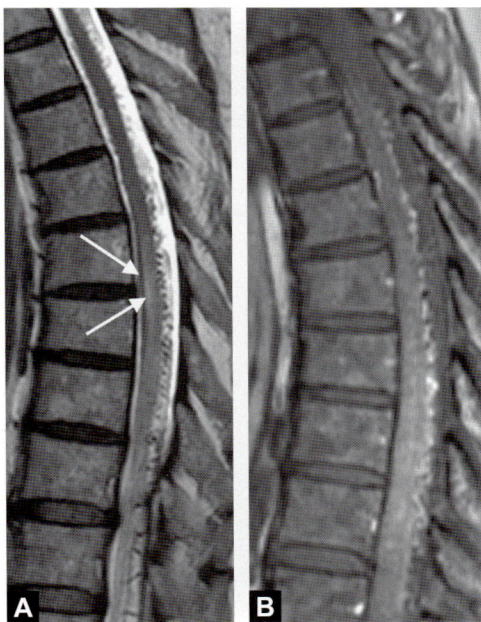

Figs. 14.10A and B: Spinal dural arteriovenous fistula. (A) Sagittal T2WI demonstrates multiple, tiny flow voids along the dorsal surface of the cord, which is normally smooth, along with mild T2-hyperintensity in the thoracic cord at T9-T10 (arrows), (B) post-gadolinium sagittal T1WI reveals multiple, enhancing serpentine veins along the dorsal surface of the spinal cord.

intra-medullary glomus type AVM, is similar in appearance on MRI to a brain AVM, typically found in the cervical or thoracic region. There is a focal nidus within the substance of the cord characterized by multiple, T2-hypointense flow voids, which is supplied by the ASA or PSA, and drains into the coronal venous plexus on the cord surface (Figs. 14.11A and B). The spinal cord is enlarged and heterogeneous in signal secondary to blood products. In type III AVM (juvenile), the rarest of all spinal AVMs, there is a large complex nidus that may have extramedullary, and even extraspinal, extension. In type IV, or perimedullary fistula, there is a direct intradural, extramedullary connection between a feeding vessel from the ASA or PSA to a spinal vein without an intervening capillary bed. On MRI, there are pronounced draining veins on the dorsal or ventral surface of the cord with T2-hyperintensity in the substance of the cord. The key differentiating features of spinal AVMs on MRI are highlighted in Table 14.3.

Spinal cord cavernous malformation (cavernoma) is an intramedullary vascular lesion typically seen in middle-aged adults with a female predominance. The spinal cord is an uncommon site for cavernomas, unlike the brain. Although typically single, multiple spinal cavernomas have been reported (familial).[27] Most frequent in the cervicothoracic region, cavernomas present as round, well-defined regions of heterogeneous signal intensity

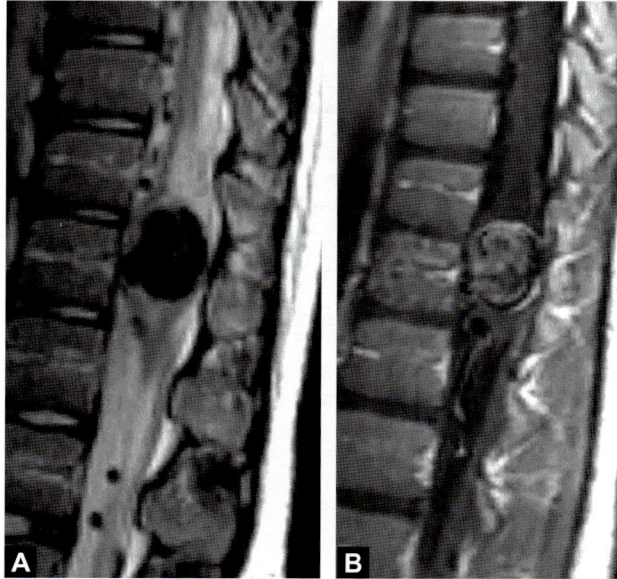

Figs. 14.11A and B: Type II spinal arteriovenous malformation (AVM). (A and B) Sagittal T2WI and post-gadolinium sagittal T1WI reveal a focal, compact intramedullary nidus in the conus medullaris characterized by multiple T2-hypointense flow voids and demonstrating enhancement.

on T1- and T2-weighted MRI sequences with possible fluid-fluid levels, and are surrounded by a T2-hypointense hemosiderin rim. The specific MRI appearance of cavernomas, described as "popcorn-like", is explained by blood products of varying ages. They may range in size from a few mm to greater than 1 cm, and there is usually no associated edema or mass effect unless there has been recent hemorrhage. On gradient-echo sequences, cavernomas demonstrate marked "blooming" due to susceptibility effects in the setting of hemosiderin deposition (Figs. 14.12A to C). The post-gadolinium magnetic resonance (MR) sequences show minimal or absent enhancement. Furthermore, angiography is usually negative ("angiographically occult"). In the setting of hematomyelia or spinal subarachnoid hemorrhage, cavernoma of the spinal cord should be strongly considered.[28]

METABOLIC CAUSES

Chief complaint/history: A 50-year-old male with Crohn's disease and gradually worsening unsteady gait, as well as numbness and tingling in both hands and feet, for 6 weeks.

Differential diagnosis:
- Subacute combined degeneration (SCD)
- Transverse myelitis
- Human immunodeficiency virus (HIV) vacuolar myelopathy.

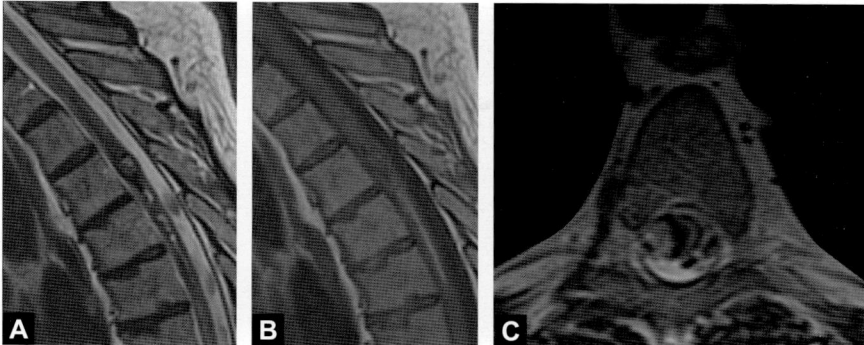

Figs. 14.12A to C: Cavernoma. (A to C) Sagittal T2WI, sagittal T1WI, and axial T2WI reveal a round, heterogeneous, eccentrically located lesion, at least partially intramedullary, within the thoracic cord at the level of T4, where there is minimal cord expansion. A T2 hypointense rim is appreciated surrounding this lesion, which is favored to represent hemosiderin, although could represent calcification. Linear, intramedullary T1/T2 hyperintense signal extends inferiorly to the level of T6, which likely represents the sequela of prior hemorrhage.

Table 14.3: Key MRI features of spinal AVMs.

Type I (SDAVF)	Prominent veins dorsal surface cord, ± cord T2-hyperintensity
Type II (intramedullary glomus)	Focal nidus in cord, heterogeneous cord signal
Type III (juvenile)	Nidus; extramedullary, extraspinal extension
Type IV AVF (perimedullary fistula)	Prominent veins dorsal or ventral surface cord

(AVM: Arteriovenous malformation; SDAVF: Spinal dural arteriovenous fistula; AVF: Arteriovenous fistula).

Discussion:

Subacute combined degeneration of the spinal cord refers to myelopathy caused by vitamin B_{12} (cobalamin) deficiency. SCD primarily affects the cervical and upper thoracic cord, although the peripheral nervous system may also be involved. The condition is characterized by demyelination and vacuolar changes in the posterior and lateral columns of the spinal cord. The most common cause of SCD in the United States is pernicious anemia, or inability to absorb vitamin B_{12} due to immune-mediated deficiency of intrinsic factor. Other causes of vitamin B_{12} deficiency include gastric surgery, malabsorption syndromes, and rarely, dietary deficiencies.

On MRI, SCD is characterized by T2-weighted hyperintensity localized to the dorsal aspect of the spinal cord in the distribution of the posterior and lateral spinal cord columns (Figs. 14.13A and B). Axial sequences demonstrate an "inverted V" or "inverted rabbit ears" of abnormal signal in the dorsal spinal cord. The signal abnormality is usually long-segment, differentiating SCD from other demyelinating disorders that may be patchy in distribution. There may be mild expansion of the cord, and post-gadolinium

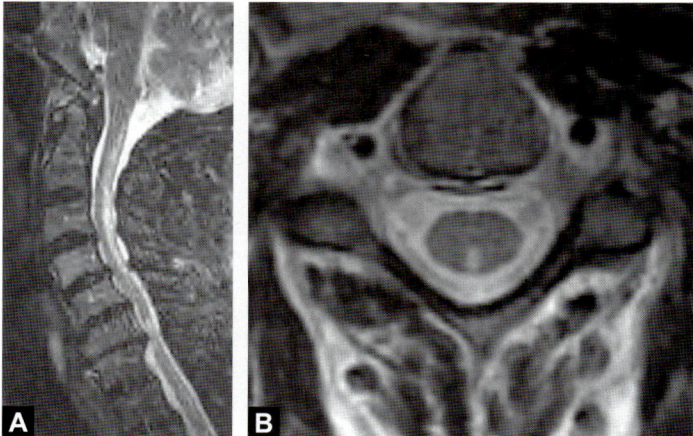

Figs. 14.13A and B: Subacute combined degeneration. (A and B) Sagittal short tau inversion recovery (STIR) and axial T2WI demonstrate selective demyelination of the dorsal spinal cord columns (T2-hyperintensity) in this patient with pernicious anemia.

Box 14.1: Degeneration of the posterior columns.
• Vitamin B$_{12}$ deficiency
• Tabes dorsalis (syphilis)
• Nitrous oxide toxicity
• Copper deficiency
• Folic acid deficiency
• HIV vacuolar myelopathy
• Multiple sclerosis

(HIV: Human immunodeficiency virus).

sequences may show mild enhancement.[29,30] Moreover, MRI of the brain may reveal T2-weighted white matter hyperintensities, which like the spinal cord findings, usually improve after treatment with vitamin B$_{12}$.[30,31] The bone marrow can be low in signal intensity on both T1- and T2-weighted sequences as a result of benign hematopoietic hyperplasia in the setting of pernicious anemia, a helpful clue in the diagnosis of SCD.

Other conditions that result in degeneration of the posterior columns of the spinal cord and present in an identical fashion on MRI include copper deficiency, folic acid deficiency, nitrous oxide toxicity, tabes dorsalis (syphilis), and vacuolar myelopathy (HIV), and as such, a comprehensive clinical history is key in distinguishing these entities (Box 14.1).

TRAUMATIC CAUSES

Chief complaint/history: A 24-year-old male with sudden onset of paraplegia after a high-speed motor vehicle accident.

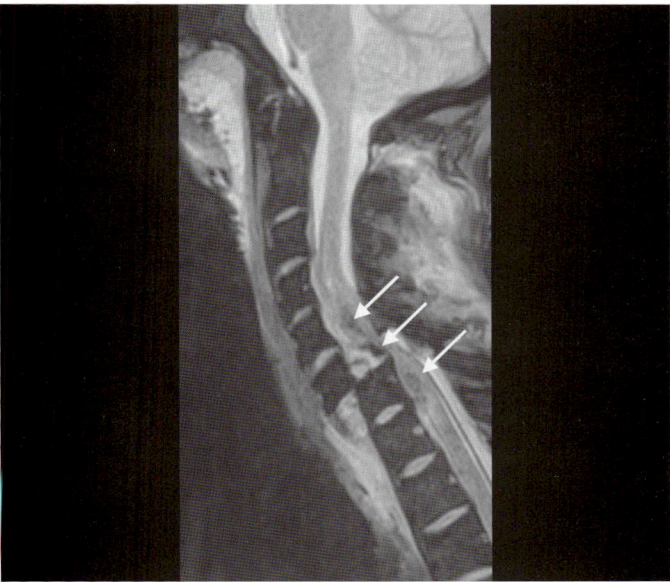

Fig. 14.14: Spinal cord injury. Sagittal gradient-echo image in a 20-year-old female after trauma demonstrates dislocation of C6 on C7 with cord compression. The cervical spinal cord is expanded with foci of signal loss from C5 to C8 (arrows), suspicious for spinal cord hemorrhage.

Differential diagnosis:
- Spinal cord edema
- Spinal cord hemorrhage
- Disk herniation with cord compression.

Discussion:
Spinal cord injury is a devastating and life-altering event. MRI provides a non-invasive means to evaluate the internal structure of the damaged spinal cord, and is able to depict parenchymal changes resulting from SCI. Moreover, MRI features of SCI are objective, well validated, and reproducible.

　　Post-traumatic spinal cord hemorrhage, or hemorrhagic contusion, refers to a focus of hemorrhage, most often hemorrhagic necrosis, in the substance of the spinal cord after an injury. The hemorrhage often occurs in the central gray matter of the spinal cord, and is situated at the point of maximal mechanical impact. On MRI, cord hemorrhage appears as a discrete focus of hypointensity on T2-weighted and gradient-echo sequences, best visualized in the midsagittal plane. Post-traumatic spinal cord hemorrhage always coexists with spinal cord edema, although the converse is not always true; cord edema is most commonly seen without hemorrhage following an injury (Fig. 14.14). Spinal cord edema is defined on MRI as an area of abnormal T2-high signal intensity, and involves a variable length of spinal cord above and below the level of injury. Relatively uniform in caliber, the normal spinal cord increases slightly in diameter in the lower cervical and lower thoracic spine. The most nondescript imaging finding associated with SCI, swelling, is defined as focal increase in caliber of the cord centered at the level of injury, and may be associated with normal to slightly hypointense signal of the cord parenchyma on T1-weighted sagittal images.[32-35] Spinal cord edema is invariably associated with some degree of cord swelling, and the length of edema is proportional to the degree of initial neurological deficit.[32,35] Although swelling denotes spinal cord dysfunction, it does not predict the extent of neurological injury.[32,35]

In the setting of trauma, MRI can also visualize subluxations and vertebral body fractures, ligamentous injury, epidural hematomas, and traumatic disk herniations.

Subacute progressive ascending myelopathy, also known as SPAM, is a rare, poorly understood complication of SCI first described by Frankel,[36] typically seen within a few weeks of injury to any part of the cord. SPAM is clinically defined as neurological impairment above the initial neurologic level of injury. It is a rare, poorly understood complication of SCI, although recovery is mostly good, unless the brain stem is involved. On MRI, there is increased T2-signal extending at least four vertebral body segments above the initial injury site with a rim of peripheral cord sparing and concomitant cord expansion.[37,38] Follow-up MRI shows near normalization of the cord changes, although there may be a focus of myelomalacia on vertebral segment above the initial injury site, as well as cord atrophy.[37,38]

REFERENCES

1. Love S. Demyelinating diseases. J Clin Pathol. 2006;59(11):1151-9.
2. Edwards MK, Farlow MR, Stevens JC. Cranial MR in spinal cord MS: diagnosing patients with isolated spinal cord symptoms. AJNR Am J Neuroradiol. 1986;7(6):1003-5.
3. Thorpe JW, Kidd D, Moseley IF, et al. Spinal MRI in patients with suspected multiple sclerosis and negative brain MRI. Brain. 1996;119(Pt 3):709-14.
4. Adams RD, Kubik CS. The morbid anatomy of the demyelinative disease. Am J Med. 1952;12(5):510-46.
5. Thielen KR, Miller GM. Multiple sclerosis of the spinal cord: magnetic resonance appearance. J Comput Assist Tomogr. 1996;20(3):434-8.
6. Rocca MA, Mastronardo G, Horsfield MA, et al. Comparison of three MR sequences for the detection of cervical cord lesions in patients with multiple sclerosis. AJNR Am J Neuroradiol. 1999;20(9):1710-6.
7. Brainin M, Neuhold A, Reisner T, et al. Changes within the "normal" cerebral white matter of multiple sclerosis patients during acute attacks and during high-dose cortisone therapy assessed by means of quantitative MRI. J Neurol Neurosurg Psychiatry. 1989;52(12):1355-9.
8. Transverse Myelitis Consortium Working Group. Proposed diagnostic criteria and nosology of acute transverse myelitis. Neurology. 2002;59(4):499-505.
9. Krishnan AV, Halmagyi GM. Acute transverse myelitis in SLE. Neurology. 2004;62(11):2087.

10. Campi A, Filippi M, Comi G, et al. Recurrent acute transverse myelopathy associated with anticardiolipin antibodies. AJNR Am J Neuroradiol. 1998;19(4): 781-6.

11. Tenembaum S, Chamoles N, Fejerman N. Acute disseminated encephalo-myelitis: a long-term follow-up study of 84 pediatric patients. Neurology. 2002;59(8):1224-31.

12. Tenembaum S, Chitnis T, Ness J, et al. Acute disseminated encephalomyelitis. Neurology. 2007;68(16 Suppl 2):S23-36.

13. Rawlings CE, Giangaspero F, Burger PC, et al. Ependymomas: a clinicopatho-logic study. Surg Neurol. 1988;29(4):271-81.

14. Goy AM, Pinto RS, Raghavendra BN, et al. Intramedullary spinal cord tumors: MR imaging, with emphasis on associated cysts. Radiology. 1986;161(2):381-6.

15. Sonneland PR, Scheithauer BW, Onofrio BM. Myxopapillary ependymoma. A clinicopathologic and immunocytochemical study of 77 cases. Cancer. 1985;56(4):883-93.

16. Farwell JR, Dohrmann GJ. Intraspinal neoplasms in children. Paraplegia. 1977;15(3):262-73.

17. Reimer R, Onofrio BM. Astrocytomas of the spinal cord in children and ado-lescents. J Neurosurg. 1985;63(5):669-75.

18. Slasky BS, Bydder GM, Niendorf HP, et al. MR imaging with gadolinium-DTPA in the differentiation of tumor, syrinx, and cyst of the spinal cord. J Comput Assist Tomogr. 1987;11(5):845-50.

19. Browne TR, Adams RD, Roberson GH. Hemangioblastoma of the spinal cord. Review and report of five cases. Arch Neurol. 1976;33(6):435-41.

20. Sze G, Krol G, Zimmerman RD, et al. Intramedullary disease of the spine: diag-nosis using gadolinium-DTPA-enhanced MR imaging. AJR Am J Roentgenol. 1988;151(6):1193-204.

21. Enomoto H, Shibata T, Ito A, et al. Multiple hemangioblastomas accompa-nied by syringomyelia in the cerebellum and the spinal cord. Surg Neurol. 1984;22(2):197-203.

22. Bornke C, Schmid G, Szymanski S, et al. Vertebral body infarction indicating midthoracic spinal stroke. Spinal Cord. 2002;40(5):244-7.

23. McCutcheon IE, Doppman JL, Oldfield EH. Microvascular anatomy of dural arteriovenous abnormalities of the spine: a microangiographic study. J Neurosurg. 1996;84(2):215-20.

24. Hirayama K, Foix C, Alajouanine T. Subacute necrotic myelitis (Foix-Alajouanine disease). Shinkei Kenkyu No Shimpo. 1970;14(1):208-25.

25. Hurst RW, Kenyon LC, Lavi E, et al. Spinal dural arteriovenous fistula: the pathology of venous hypertensive myelopathy. Neurology. 1995;45(7):1309-13.

26. Hurst RW, Grossman RI. Peripheral spinal cord hypointensity on T2-weighted MR images: a reliable imaging sign of venous hypertensive myelopathy. AJNR Am J Neuroradiol. 2000;21(4):781-6.

27. Lee KS, Spetzler RF. Spinal cord cavernous malformation in a patient with familial intracranial cavernous malformations. Neurosurgery. 1990;26(5): 877-80.

28. Ueda S, Saito A, Inomori S, et al. Cavernous angioma of the cauda equina pro-ducing subarachnoid hemorrhage. Case report. J Neurosurg. 1987;66(1):134-6.

29. Larner AJ, Zeman AZ, Allen CM, et al. MRI appearances in subacute com-bined degeneration of the spinal cord due to vitamin B12 deficiency. J Neurol Neurosurg Psychiatry. 1997;62(1):99-100.

30. Ravina B, Loevner LA, Bank W. MR findings in subacute combined degeneration of the spinal cord: a case of reversible cervical myelopathy. AJR Am J Roentgenol. 2000;174(3):863-5.
31. Stojsavljevic N, Levic Z, Drulovic J, et al. A 44-month clinical-brain MRI follow-up in a patient with B12 deficiency. Neurology. 1997;49(3):878-81.
32. Flanders AE, Schaefer DM, Doan HT, et al. Acute cervical spine trauma: correlation of MR imaging findings with degree of neurologic deficit. Radiology. 1990;177(1):25-33.
33. Kulkarni MV, McArdle CB, Kopanicky D, et al. Acute spinal cord injury: MR imaging at 1.5 T. Radiology. 1987;164(3):837-43.
34. Kalfas I, Wilberger J, Goldberg A, et al. Magnetic resonance imaging in acute spinal cord trauma. Neurosurgery. 1988;23(3):295-9.
35. Schaefer DM, Flanders A, Northrup BE, et al. Magnetic resonance imaging of acute cervical spine trauma. Correlation with severity of neurologic injury. Spine. 1989;14(10):1090-5.
36. Frankel HL. Ascending cord lesion in the early stages following spinal injury. Paraplegia. 1969;7(2):111-8.
37. Planner AC, Pretorius PM, Graham A, et al. Subacute progressive ascending myelopathy following spinal cord injury: MRI appearances and clinical presentation. Spinal Cord. 2008;46(2):140-4.
38. Yablon IG, Ordia J, Mortara R, et al. Acute ascending myelopathy of the spine. Spine. 1989;14(10):1084-9.

Index

Note: Page numbers followed by f refer to figure and t refer to table.